Mental Disorders.

Awareness and Help.

For parents, Guardians, and Caregivers

Written By

Jorge A Garcia

The author of this book does not dispense medical advice or prescribe the use of any technique as a form of treatment for physical, emotional, or medical problems without the advice of a physician, either directly or indirectly. The author's intent is only to offer information of a general nature to help you in your quest for emotional, physical, and spiritual well-being. If you use any of the information in this book for yourself, the author and the publisher assume no responsibility for your actions.

This book is not intended to substitute the medical advice of physicians. The reader should regularly consult a physician in matters relating to their health, particularly concerning symptoms that may require diagnosis or medical attention.

This book is for educational information and does not constitute medical advice. Please consult a medical or health professional before you begin any exercise, nutrition, or supplementation program or if you have questions about your health.

Some names and identifying details have been changed to protect the privacy of individuals.

I have tried to recreate events, locales, and conversations from my memories of them. To maintain their anonymity, I have sometimes changed the names of individuals and places. I may have changed some identifying characteristics and details, such as physical properties, occupations, and areas of residence.

Authored by a fellow concerned parent, this guide is written in an easy-to-understand manner (no medical jargon). So, even if you've felt lost in your attempts to comprehend your child's struggles, let this guide bring you the clarity you desire.

Contents

Introduction

The COVID-19 pandemic caused irrefutable damage globally. There's no debate about this.

Millions of lives were lost, economies were shattered, and the entire world came to a standstill. Yet, within this devastating physical impact, a more insidious consequence emerged—the silent erosion of mental health, particularly among our young population. The trauma inflicted by the pandemic through the disruption of their education, means of livelihood, families, lives lost, and more is enough to shake the foundation of their mental well-being – if it shook ours as adults, how about them?

25% - this marks the global increase in mental health issues after the Covid 19 pandemic. But the sad reality is that this number only scratches the surface of the absolute magnitude of the problem. Countless cases remain undocumented and untreated, contributing to a grim rise in suicide rates, especially among the younger generation.

Why We Wrote This Book?

So, we can safeguard our children's mental well-being as parents and caregivers.

So, we can identify the signs that indicate all might not be well and extend a helping hand to guide them out of the consuming world of mental health problems.

Your child, whether a newborn, an infant, a preschooler, or even a teenager, depends entirely on you as their parent or caregiver for physical, emotional, psychological, and financial support. So, while we may feel like mental health is outside of the scope of parenting, the truth is quite the opposite.

Consider it this way: if your child faces mental health challenges, picture how overwhelming their world must be. Their everyday life is plagued with confusing and sometimes intense emotions and situations, and this is where the knowledge you learn in this book will play a vital role. It will help you offer understanding, empathy, and support they desperately need.

While some mental and behavioral disorders can be easily identified at birth or a few years later, some develop over time and can be hard to pinpoint if you are not keen enough.

This book will cover both, including some of the most prevalent pediatric mental disorders, their symptoms, causes, challenges, and steps for treatment.

As you read this book, I urge you to keep an open heart and a receptive mind. The goal is not merely to teach you but to help you foster a deeper connection with your child as you understand a little bit about their world and experiences.

This book is not just a collection of facts; it contains essential information about pediatric mental health issues. Instead, it is a guide and a companion for all who seek to comprehend their child's emotional world.

So, if you are a parent, a caregiver, or a loved one to someone with a child struggling with a mental ailment, this book is for you.

Let's get started.

Chapter 1: Introduction to Pediatric Psychiatric Disorders

This chapter provides a foundational understanding of child psychiatric disorders, emphasizing their significance for parents and caregivers. By defining these conditions and stressing the importance of parental awareness, it aims to promote informed and supportive approaches to pediatric mental health.

Definition of Child Psychiatric Disorders:

Child psychiatric disorders, or pediatric mental health disorders, encompass various conditions affecting children and adolescents' emotional, cognitive, and behavioral well-being. These conditions manifest in diverse ways, including mood disturbances, thought process issues, and difficulties in interpersonal interactions.

Diverse Range of Conditions:

This section offers a comprehensive definition of child psychiatric disorders, highlighting the diversity within this category. It mentions specific conditions like anxiety disorders, attention-deficit/hyperactivity disorder (ADHD), depression, and autism spectrum disorders. It also underscores how these disorders may present differently in children than adults, emphasizing the need for specialized understanding.

Evolution of Understanding Child Psychiatric Disorders:

Understanding the historical context of child psychiatric disorders helps us appreciate the transformation from superstition and stigma to scientific comprehension and empathy. Over time, there has been a significant shift in how society perceives and treats these disorders.

Ancient Beliefs and Supernatural Explanations:

In ancient times, behaviors now recognized as indicative of child psychiatric disorders were often attributed to supernatural causes such as curses or evil spirits. Children displaying unusual behavior were isolated or subjected to exorcisms due to a lack of understanding.

Emergence of Medical Perspectives:

In the 18th and 19th centuries, medical professionals started acknowledging neurobiological factors as contributors to these disorders. However, treatments remained rudimentary, often involving isolation or restraint.

From Moral Failings to Medical Conditions:

The 20th century saw a transformation in how child psychiatric disorders were viewed. They shifted from being seen as moral failings to being understood as medical conditions requiring compassionate care. Psychological theories gained prominence during this period.

Integration of Psychological and Biological Factors:

Advancements in medical science and psychology have led to a more integrated understanding of

these disorders. Researchers identified the roles of genetics, brain chemistry, and environmental factors, paving the way for targeted interventions.

Shaping Modern Approaches:

Today, our understanding of child psychiatric disorders continues to evolve. Interdisciplinary collaboration and ongoing research have helped identify risk factors, develop effective treatments, and reduce stigma. Schools, families, and communities now recognize the importance of comprehensive support for children's mental well-being.

COVID-19's Impact on Children's Psychiatric Disorders:

The COVID-19 pandemic has disrupted students' lives, with school closures affecting academic development and mental health care access. Schools traditionally provided mental health services for many students, making access challenging during closures, especially for vulnerable groups. Policymakers must address these disruptions and improve long-term mental health services for children.

Promoting Empathy and Informed Care:

The historical trajectory from supernatural explanations to scientific understanding highlights the importance of knowledge and empathy. Understanding this history allows us to advocate for informed and compassionate care for children and adolescents with psychiatric disorders.

In the upcoming chapters, we will delve deeper into specific disorders, their symptoms, and evidence-based treatment approaches. This historical context serves as a reminder of the progress made and the ongoing work needed to enhance the lives of young individuals with psychiatric disorders.

Chapter 2: Trauma and Stressor-Related Disorders

Post-Traumatic Stress Disorder (PTSD) and acute stress disorder

Post-Traumatic Stress Disorder (PTSD) is a challenging and distressing mental health condition that can affect adults and children. When children experience or witness a traumatic event, their emotional and psychological well-being can be profoundly impacted. This introduction delves into the unique aspects of PTSD in children, exploring its causes, symptoms, and the importance of early intervention and support.

Childhood is typically considered a time of innocence and carefree joy, but unfortunately, not all children can grow up in such an environment. For some, life takes an unexpected turn when they encounter traumatic experiences that leave lasting scars on their minds and hearts. PTSD in children is a poignant reminder of the vulnerability of young minds and the need for compassionate understanding and effective treatment.

How common is PTSD?

Traumatic Events Happen to Many Kids: It turns out that about 1 in 4 children and teenagers go through something challenging or scary during their childhood or teenage years. These events are called "traumatic."

Not Everyone Gets PTSD: The good news is that most kids who experience these challenging events don't end up with PTSD, a particular condition that can happen after trauma.

Different Kinds of PTSD: This condition has a couple of different versions. One is called "acute stress disorder," which can affect about 1 in 5 to 1 in 2 kids after trauma. The other is the full-blown "childhood PTSD," which affects around 1 in 6 kids who've been through trauma.

Boys and Girls Can Be Affected Differently: The chances of getting PTSD can differ for boys and girls, and it also depends on the type of trauma. For example, girls who've experienced trauma involving people they know are more likely to get PTSD, with 1 in 3 developing it. Boys who've experienced different types of traumas have a lower chance, around 1 in 12.

More Girls, More Risk: Girls experience traumatic events and PTSD more often than boys.

Factors That Raise the Risk: Some things can make it more likely for a child to get PTSD after a challenging event. These include how bad or how long the trauma was, how close the child was to it, if they could have been hurt, and if the trauma involves someone they know being violent.

Also, if a child had problems with anxiety before the trauma, it could increase the risk.

Disasters and PTSD: In situations like disasters (like earthquakes or floods), apprehensive kids who panic during the event or don't leave the dangerous area in time are more at risk of getting PTSD.

So, to put it simply, many kids go through tough times, but not all get PTSD. Girls are more likely to get it, especially if the trauma involves people they know. The type of trauma and how bad it was also played a role, along with other factors like anxiety and how kids react during disasters.

What Causes PTSD in Kids?

PTSD (Post-Traumatic Stress Disorder) usually happens after a child goes through something scary or traumatic. This event is called the "traumatic event."

Certain types of traumatic events, like ones where a child gets hurt or sees violence, might make it more likely for a child to get PTSD. These events are significantly linked to something called.
"Acute stress disorder" is like an early form of PTSD.

Some kids might be more likely to get PTSD if they've had a tough life before the traumatic event, like problems in their family or other mental health issues.

Sometimes, even if a child has no issues before, a bad traumatic event can still lead to PTSD.

The Complicated Start of PTSD:

Starting to have PTSD is quite complicated. It involves changes in hormones (which control our bodies), genes, thoughts, feelings, and how we interact with others.

When children go through abuse or neglect (not being taken care of properly), it can affect their thinking, development, and how they react to things because of brain changes.

How PTSD progresses in children

The course (how it progresses) and prognosis (what might happen in the future) of PTSD in children can vary. Some studies suggest that about half of kids with PTSD symptoms no longer have them after six months without treatment. However, other research shows that some children continue to experience these symptoms over time.

Certain factors can influence whether PTSD symptoms persist or improve. These factors include being a girl, experiencing a sense of disconnection during the traumatic event, and coming from a family with a lower income. In some cases, having symptoms like feeling detached from reality and being overly alert can predict the development of full-blown PTSD.

After a traumatic event, things like losing their home, being separated from friends and family, or losing loved ones can make PTSD symptoms worse. A loving and supportive family and a safe environment can help ease these symptoms.

Kids with PTSD may also experience other issues like anxiety, depression, trouble concentrating, and a lack of motivation. This can make it hard for them to do well in school and feel hopeful about the future.

If some children don't receive treatment, their outlook might not be positive. Untreated childhood PTSD can lead to problems in adulthood, such as suicide attempts, major depression, feeling disconnected from reality, and daily struggles. Childhood trauma, like abuse, can also increase the risk of mental health issues in adulthood, especially for women.

Role of parents and teachers in identifying a child with PTSD

When children show significant changes in their behavior or emotions, it's essential to consider the possibility of acute stress disorder or PTSD, even if we don't know about a specific traumatic event. It's not always easy for children to talk about what they've been through or how they're feeling, so we need to look for signs. Talking to different people who know the child, like parents, teachers, or caregivers, is innovative because sometimes kids might only share some things with one person. Sometimes, caregivers may be unaware of what the child is going through or may find it hard to talk about it.

The child's history and experiences can also provide clues, and tools like rating scales and checklists can help professionals assess their symptoms. Observations from teachers about changes in the child's behavior or school performance can also be constructive in figuring things out.

Treatment for a child with PTSD

Identifying children who might be at risk for PTSD early after a traumatic event is important because it can help prevent them from experiencing long-term emotional distress. This is especially crucial when something big, like a natural disaster, affects many kids.

One way to help them is through the Child and Family Traumatic Stress Intervention (CFTSI) program. It involves four sessions where kids learn about what they're going through, how to relax, and ways to cope with their feelings. This approach is more effective than only regular care in preventing PTSD from getting worse. So, quick identification and the right help can make a significant difference for these children.

When it comes to helping children with PTSD, there are diverse ways to do it. The treatment should be sensitive to the child's age and culture and consider how trauma affects the brain. It's essential to involve parents or caregivers, focus on making the child feel safe, and address the things that remind them of the trauma.

One practical approach is called Trauma-focused Cognitive-Behavioral Therapy (TF-CBT). It involves several steps, like educating the child and their parents, teaching relaxation techniques, and helping them manage their feelings and thoughts about the trauma. They also work on creating a story about the trauma and learning how to deal with memories of it.

There are other treatments, like group therapy in schools, improving relationships between young kids and their parents, and specialized medicines for specific situations. It's important to recognize if parents or caregivers also need help with their trauma because it can affect the child, too.

In some cases, web-based programs have been developed to make it easier for kids to get treatment. The main goal is to help these children heal and feel better after experiencing a traumatic event.

Psychotherapy before medication

When treating PTSD in kids, the first choice is usually psychotherapy, not medication. Medication might be considered if the child has another condition that requires it, if they're in immediate danger, or if their symptoms are severe and not getting better with therapy.

For medication, there's limited evidence that certain drugs like selective serotonin reuptake inhibitors, propranolol, clonidine, prazosin (for nightmares), morphine (for pain in burn victims), or risperidone can help, but it's not super strong evidence. Because of this, medication should only be used when your doctor says it's needed.

Chapter 3: Eating and Feeding Disorders

Anorexia Nervosa

Anorexia nervosa is a severe eating disorder where a person intentionally tries to lose weight by restricting their food intake or using extreme measures. They may have a distorted view of their body shape and size, thinking they are much larger than they are. Some people with anorexia deny how dangerous their weight loss is.

People with anorexia are often obsessed with food and their appearance. In severe cases, they might even seem delusional. They're afraid of gaining weight, even if they are already underweight. It's important to note that they don't lose their appetite; they are just terrified of putting on weight.

There are two main types of anorexia:

Restricting Type: People with this type severely limit their food intake, often by dieting, fasting, or exercising excessively.

Binge-Eating/Purging Type: Here, individuals eat substantial amounts of food in a short time (binge) and then try to get rid of it, typically through vomiting or using laxatives.
(purging).

As the body starves, it leads to more psychological symptoms. Anorexia can cause social withdrawal, irritability, and a lack of interest in things that used to bring joy. Some people might experience symptoms like major depression, such as feeling helpless and worthless.

Depression can make it difficult to function well in school, with friends, or at home. People with anorexia often want to control their eating habits and those around them. They might become highly focused on academic achievement and exercise.

In some cases, individuals with anorexia also have obsessive-compulsive disorder (OCD), which means they have intrusive, distressing thoughts and engage in repetitive behaviors.

Remember, anorexia is a serious condition that can have severe health consequences. If you or someone you know is struggling with an eating disorder, it's essential to seek help from a medical professional as soon as possible.

How common in which age group

Most individuals with anorexia nervosa (AN) are female, estimated to affect about 0.3% to 0.7% of teenage girls in the United States. It's rare for AN to begin before puberty. The highest number of new cases occurs in people aged 14 to 24. There are also less severe forms of eating disorders that are more common. AND is found in Western industrialized countries, and societal and social factors influence its prevalence. In boys, minority groups, and

non-Western countries, AN is less common, but its rates are increasing.

Factors Associated with Anorexia Nervosa (AN):

AN has connections to biological, psychological, and environmental factors, but it's unclear if they cause it.

Genetics play a role; if a close family member has an eating disorder, you're more likely to have one.

It's hard to tell what's genetic and what's due to the environment.

People with AN often have issues in various parts of their lives: psychologically, physically, academically, and socially.

They often become unhappy with their bodies during puberty. Dieting is seen to feel better and gain control.

People with AN are often perfectionistic and detail-oriented and might have a rigid way of thinking.

Societal beauty ideals, peer pressure, and specific activities can increase AN risk.

Family Dynamics and AN:

Some research has focused on family dynamics, like parents being too involved or not setting clear boundaries.

However, these characteristics can also be found in families where eating disorders don't develop.

So, it needs to be clarified if family dynamics directly cause AN.

Challenges and complications that children with AN face challenges

AN usually begins during adolescence, around ages 14 to 18.
This is when your body is growing fast, and you naturally gain weight and your shape changes.
While it's less common, some kids may develop AN or unhealthy eating habits before puberty.
These habits can include avoiding certain foods, being unhappy with their appearance, trying diets that aren't right for them, overeating at times, having rituals around meals, or being very fussy about what they eat.
Sometimes, the first sign of trouble is when they focus on dieting. In one study, over half of the girls thought they were overweight when only 15% were. So, it shows how body image concerns can start early.

Complications

Common Physiological Effects:

AN often leads to physical health problems.

Some of these problems can be profoundly serious, requiring a person to be hospitalized. Long-Term Course of AN:

AN tends to last a long time and doesn't go away on its own. People with AN may continue to have symptoms like being too thin for their age and height, worrying too much about their weight or how they look, delays in puberty, missed periods, and difficulties in social and romantic relationships.

Factors Influencing Outcome:

The outlook for someone with AN can be affected by how long they've had the illness, how much weight they've lost, and how well they get along with others.

Teens with AN usually have a better chance of getting better and fewer chances of dying than adults.

Risk of Death:

AN can be profoundly serious, with a risk of death.

About 5% to 7% of people with AN may die from health problems related to the illness. Sadly, up to half of these deaths can be because of suicide.

Impact of Other Mental Health Issues:

Having other mental health problems alongside AN can make the outlook worse.

Many people with AN might get better, but not entirely, especially when they also have other mental health issues.

Identifying a child with AN

The interview with someone suspected of having AN should cover various aspects.

Information like when the eating disorder started, how it has progressed, the highest and lowest weight, and the importance the person feels most comfortable with.

Understanding their daily eating habits, including what they eat, when they eat, and any use of laxatives, emetics, diuretics, or exercise to control their weight.

Even though individuals with AN often try to hide their behaviors, they might unintentionally reveal essential details during this discussion.

Family members can sometimes provide additional insights, although individuals with AN may not share their symptoms with their families.

Family Evaluation:

Evaluating the family is crucial when treating you're loved ones with AN.

This involves asking family members about their thoughts on the illness and its origins.

Exploring previous attempts at home-based treatments can reveal family dynamics and how everyone perceives the issue and potential solutions.

Looking into the family's eating or weight history might uncover patterns that the child or adolescent has adopted.

A family history of mental health issues may also offer clues about potential diagnoses for the patient.

A complete history, physical examination, and routine laboratory studies are necessary to rule out other psychiatric or medical causes for weight or appetite loss.

Bulimia Nervosa: This eating disorder involves episodes of overeating followed by compensatory behaviors like vomiting or excessive exercise, whereas individuals with AN primarily restrict food intake.

Avoidant/Restrictive Food Intake Disorder (ARFID): ARFID is characterized by limited food preferences or avoidance of certain foods due to sensory sensitivities, aversions, or other factors. Unlike AN, it's not driven by a desire to lose weight or body image concerns.

Body Dysmorphic Disorder (BDD): Individuals with BDD obsessively focus on perceived flaws in their appearance, including body shape and size. While body image concerns are present in AN, BDD is primarily centered around a distorted view of specific body parts.

Depression: Symptoms of depression can overlap with AN, including changes in appetite, weight loss, and low self-esteem. However, depression doesn't involve the same intense fear of gaining weight or restrictive eating behaviors seen in AN.

Generalized Anxiety Disorder (GAD): GAD may feature excessive worry about body weight and shape, but it lacks the specific dietary restrictions and weight loss goals of AN.

Obsessive-Compulsive Disorder (OCD): OCD can involve body image or weight obsessions. However, the compulsions in OCD typically differ from the eating-related behaviors seen in AN.

Medical Conditions: Certain conditions, such as hyperthyroidism or gastrointestinal disorders, can lead to unintentional weight loss. It's essential to rule out these underlying medical causes before diagnosing AN.

Substance Abuse: Substance abuse, particularly stimulant drugs, can suppress appetite and lead to weight loss. This should be considered when assessing individuals with AN-like symptoms.

Autism Spectrum Disorder (ASD): Individuals with ASD may have rigid eating patterns and food preferences, but these behaviors are usually related to sensory sensitivities and repetitive behaviors rather than body image concerns.

Normal Variation in Eating Behaviors: Some people may have irregular eating habits or periods of dietary restriction without meeting the criteria for AN. These variations may not indicate a clinical disorder.

A thorough evaluation by a mental health professional is essential to differentiate AN from these other conditions and make an accurate diagnosis.

Treating a child with AN

Comprehensive Approach:

Focus on returning to regular eating habits.

Acceptance and Weight Gain:

Start by acknowledging the disorder and achieving a healthy weight.

Severe cases might require hospitalization, especially if the patient has Lost over 25% of the ideal body weight.
Rapid and severe weight loss.

Hypothermia (extremely low body temperature). Low heart rate. Severe dehydration or electrolyte imbalances. Abnormal heart rhythms.

Target Weight:

Aim for a target weight within 90% of the ideal body weight. Achieve this through gradual weight gain:

One pound per week as an outpatient. 2–3 pounds per week if hospitalized.

Avoid rapid weight gain to prevent refeeding syndrome, a dangerous condition.

Medical Team:

Involve a primary care physician and a dietitian experienced in eating disorders.

Psychotherapy:

Use therapy alongside refeeding to address underlying psychological factors. Understand that just forcing weight gain isn't enough.

Avoid Extreme Measures:

Appetite stimulants aren't recommended.

Tube or intravenous feeding is for emergencies due to potential risks and patient resistance.

Comprehensive Plan:

Develop a complete treatment plan that explores the psychological aspects of AN.

Remember, AN treatment is complex and requires a multidisciplinary approach for the best results.

Family-Based Treatment (FBT) for Anorexia Nervosa in a nutshell.

Strong Empirical Support:

FBT, known as the Maudsley model, is a highly effective treatment.

Family Impact:

Families are affected by eating disorders but don't always have pre-existing problems. Don't assume the family is to blame.

Psychoeducational Programs:

Programs to educate families extensively help with treatment. These can be individual or group sessions.

Family Involvement:

Family participation in treatment is crucial.

It emphasizes that parents are part of the solution, not the cause.

Parent-Focused Treatment (PFT):

A modification of FBT is where the therapist works with parents while a nurse monitors the patient.

Based on a study, PFT is more efficient at restoring weight in adolescents with AN.

Other strategies used to treat AN

Individual Psychotherapy:

The second choice may be needed if families can't participate.

Adolescent Focused Therapy (AFT) and Cognitive-Behavioral Therapy (CBT):

Proven to work in AN treatment.

CBT focuses on changing harmful beliefs about food, appearance, and control.

Cognitive-behavioral techniques like food diaries are helpful, especially post-weight restoration.

Interpersonal Psychotherapy:

Applicable after normalizing eating patterns.

Older patients do well with individual therapy; younger ones benefit more from family therapy.

Medication Use:

Limited evidence supporting medication for AN.

Atypical antipsychotics and SSRIs (selective serotonin reuptake inhibitors) are ineffective. SSRIs may help with anxiety and depression, but only after weight stabilizes.

Medications are typically reserved for comorbid conditions or when other treatments fail.

Your care physician will advise what's better for the patient.

Bulimia Nervosa

Bulimia nervosa, often called bulimia, is a severe eating disorder that can affect children and adolescents. It's characterized by recurring episodes of binge eating, where a person consumes.

Substantial amounts of food while feeling out of control. These episodes occur at least once a week for three months or more.

After binge eating, individuals with bulimia often use compensatory behaviors to "undo" their consumed calories. This can include excessive exercise, strict fasting, or induced vomiting. They might also use laxatives, enemas, diuretics, or other medications to control their weight.

Binge eating is typically done secretly and can initially feel pleasurable, relieving negative emotions or stress. However, the individual often experiences self-critical thoughts afterward, feeling that their eating is out of control.

One of the key features of bulimia is that individuals are often of average weight or only slightly above or below their ideal weight. Despite this, they have an intense preoccupation with the body shape and weight, which significantly influences their self-image.

Bulimia nervosa can have severe physical and emotional consequences, making it crucial for parents and caregivers to be aware of the signs and seek professional help if they suspect their child may be struggling with this disorder. Early intervention and support are essential for
effective treatment and recovery.

Understanding the Epidemiology of Bulimia Nervosa in Children

Bulimia nervosa (often called bulimia) is more common than anorexia nervosa (another eating disorder), but it's still a serious concern, especially among young people. The tricky part is that it's not always easy to spot, and studies are trying to figure out how common it is, facing some challenges.

We know that about half the time, bulimia starts before a person turns 18. So, it can affect teenagers and even younger kids.

Binge eating, which means devouring much food and feeling like you can't control it, happens quite often among teenagers. But only a smaller number have all the signs and symptoms needed for a bulimia diagnosis.

In the United States, about 1% to 2% of teenage girls and 0.5% of adolescent boys met the criteria for bulimia nervosa based on the older diagnostic rules (DSM-IV). It's important to note that boys can also have bulimia, although it's less common than in girls.

Some groups of people have a higher risk of bulimia. For example, ballet dancers and

elite athletes in sports that emphasize being very thin can be more prone to it. Also, people with bulimia often have other challenges, like using drugs or alcohol, feeling anxious or depressed, or dealing with post-traumatic stress disorder (PTSD).

Interestingly, bulimia is often linked to higher socioeconomic status, which means people from well-off families might be more at risk. Most of the time, people with bulimia are white or Hispanic. However, there are signs that rates are increasing among African Americans, even though it's still less common than in white or Latina populations.

Additionally, many teenage girls are trying to lose weight through dieting. Somewhere between 40% and 60% of them are dieting, especially those from wealthier families. Sadly, some might use unhealthy methods like making themselves vomit or taking diet pills and diuretics.

This dieting can increase the risk of developing eating disorders, including bulimia.

What causes BN?

Etiology (Causes) of Bulimia Nervosa in Children

Bulimia nervosa (bulimia) and anorexia nervosa (anorexia) often show overlapping symptoms in many patients.

Around 50% of those with anorexia will develop bulimic behaviors, and up to 25% of people with bulimia might start behaving more like they have anorexia.

There's a hint that genes play a role because if someone has an identical twin with bulimia, they also have a higher chance of having it.

Family history can matter, especially if there's a history of obesity, depression, or alcoholism.

Experiencing sexual or physical abuse can make children more vulnerable to various mental health issues, but it doesn't necessarily lead to eating disorders like bulimia. These disorders are more complex and involve multiple factors.

Prognosis (Outlook) of Bulimia Nervosa in Children

It often starts with dieting, and then binge eating becomes a response to food restriction. Binge-eating is seen as immoral behavior, leading to sadness and self-criticism.
To undo the binge, they start dieting again, with a lot of exercise or purging (like vomiting).

This cycle maintains bulimia and depression. It can also lead to semi-starvation, which makes mood problems worse.

Many adolescents with bulimia have thoughts of suicide (53%), and some even attempt it (35%). Relapse (the problem coming back) is standard, with 30% to 50% rates in 6 months to 6 years. Improvement can continue for 10 to 15 years.

Some risk factors for relapse include vomiting and using alcohol or drugs. When they start treatment, those with milder symptoms tend to do better.

If anxiety or mood disorders are also present, it's more likely that eating problems will continue. Unfortunately, no apparent factors predict who will get better with treatment.

The mortality rate for bulimia is around 5%, but this is rare.

Challenges and Complications of Bulimia Nervosa in Children

Bulimia can create significant problems in a person's life, like spending lots of time and money on food and binge-eating and purging.

It can make it harder to do well in school and have good relationships with friends.

People with bulimia might also have other issues like anxiety, depression, PTSD, and using drugs.

If someone has another medical problem and bulimia, it can make things even more dangerous.

There's a risk of suicide or severe health problems, especially if bulimia lasts long or someone is bingeing or purging daily.

Treatment for Bulimia Nervosa in Children

The main goals of treatment are to stop the cycle of binge eating and purging, develop healthy eating habits, and learn new ways to deal with emotions and challenging situations.

Treatment usually starts with ensuring the person eats regular, balanced meals to prevent intense hunger that triggers binge eating. Most kids with bulimia who maintain an average weight don't need to be in the hospital.

Hospitalization might be necessary if the person feels very suicidal, has trouble controlling their eating and purging, has unstable health, or doesn't get better with outpatient treatment. In the hospital, a plan can be made, and activities and privileges can depend on eating regular meals and not purging.

A special family-based treatment works for bulimia in teenagers, and cognitive-behavioral therapy (CBT) is highly effective in adults. CBT can also benefit teenagers from families with many conflicts.

Medications aren't typically recommended for teenagers with bulimia, but sometimes, antidepressants can help with other mental health issues. A drug called fluoxetine has been used in some cases, but more research is needed.

Avoidant/Restrictive Food Intake Disorder (ARFID)

ARFID, also known as avoidant/restrictive food intake disorder, is a distinct eating disorder that primarily affects children and adolescents. In contrast to other eating disorders like anorexia nervosa or bulimia nervosa, ARFID is not always accompanied by worries about one's

appearance or a desire to reduce weight. Instead, the excessive avoidance or limitation of

foods or food groups, which results in a restricted and highly selected diet, distinguishes ARFID. This condition may significantly affect a child's physical health, development, and general well-being. Identifying and treating this disease in children requires understanding ARFID and its intricacies.

How common is ARFID?

Regarding Avoidant/Restrictive Food Intake Disorder (ARFID) in children, little information is available regarding its prevalence in the general population. However, exciting insights have been gained from clinical settings where children seek help for this disorder.

In one eating disorders clinic catering to young patients aged 8 to 18, it was observed that approximately 14% of these individuals were diagnosed with ARFID. This diagnosis indicated they exhibited extreme pickiness with their food choices or had severely limited diets.

Remarkably, in this clinic, more boys than girls were found to have ARFID, which differs from the typical gender distribution seen in other eating disorders. Additionally, these children with ARFID tended to be younger and frequently presented with concurrent medical or

anxiety-related conditions.

In another clinical context, focusing on gastrointestinal issues, approximately 1.5% of the children exhibited symptoms aligning with ARFID. This suggests that ARFID affects eating habits and can have implications for the digestive system. Once again, a higher proportion of boys than girls was noted among those with ARFID.

What causes ARFID?

Many kids who end up with ARFID have been fussy eaters for a long time, even when they were young. Some patterns are common reasons behind ARFID in children.

One typical pattern is just not being interested in food. These kids might need to get more excited about meals or try new foods.

Another pattern is when children have a limited diet because of issues with their senses. For example, they might find certain textures or tastes unpleasant, so they avoid foods with those characteristics.

The least common pattern is when kids have a bad or scary experience related to food, like choking or getting sick, which makes them afraid of certain foods.

So, ARFID can develop from these different patterns, but they all involve having an adamant time with eating.

Why is it essential to tell ARFID apart from others?

It's vital to tell ARFID apart from other conditions because they have different causes and effects on a person's health. Here's why:

Medical Conditions: Sometimes, kids might not eat well because they have medical problems,
Like issues with their stomach or digestion, these conditions need different types of treatment, so doctors need to figure out if it's a medical problem or ARFID.

Not About Weight: Unlike anorexia, where people want to lose weight and are unhappy with their bodies, ARFID isn't about that. Kids with ARFID aren't trying to lose weight or feeling bad about their bodies.

Nutrition and Health: ARFID can affect a child's nutrition and overall health. They might not be getting all the essential nutrients they need, which can lead to problems like being underweight or having nutritional deficiencies.

Treating a child with ARFID

Children with ARFID with severe nutritional problems might need treatment in the hospital. But for those who can be treated at home, a team of experts, like doctors and therapists, will work with the child and their family to help them with their fussy eating and food-related fears. The treatment will depend on why the child is struggling with eating, and it may involve different types of therapy to address their specific issues.

Chapter 4: Anxiety Disorders

Generalized Anxiety Disorder

Generalized Anxiety Disorder (GAD) in children is a mental health condition characterized by excessive and persistent worry or anxiety about various aspects of their life. Unlike everyday concerns that come and go, GAD involves constant and overwhelming feelings of unease, often without a specific cause. Here's a description of GAD in children:

Persistent Worry: Children with GAD tend to worry excessively about everyday things such as school, friendships, family, and safety. They may worry about things that might happen in the future, even if the likelihood is low.

Physical Symptoms: GAD can manifest physically, causing symptoms like restlessness, muscle tension, headaches, stomachaches, and trouble sleeping. These physical symptoms often result from ongoing stress and anxiety.

Perfectionism: Children with GAD may set high standards for themselves and worry about not meeting them, leading to perfectionism. They may seek constant reassurance from adults.

Difficulty Concentrating: Excessive worry can make it hard for children to focus on tasks, leading to problems in school and other activities. They may become easily distracted.

Avoidance: To cope with their anxiety, children with GAD might avoid situations or activities that trigger their worries. This can limit their social interactions and experiences.

Physical Complaints: Some children may express their anxiety through physical complaints like headaches or stomachaches, which may not have an underlying medical cause.

Need for Reassurance: Children with GAD may repeatedly seek reassurance from parents or caregivers, asking for confirmation that things will be okay.

Impact on Daily Life: GAD can significantly impact a child's daily life, affecting their academic performance, relationships, and overall well-being.

Co-Occurrence: GAD often co-occurs with other anxiety disorders or conditions like depression, making diagnosis and treatment more complex.

Recognizing the signs of GAD in children and seeking professional help is essential. Early intervention and appropriate treatment, which may include therapy and, in some cases, medication, can help children manage their anxiety and lead more fulfilling lives.

How common

It's normal for kids to feel anxious from time to time. However, Generalized Anxiety Disorder (GAD) is a condition where this anxiety becomes intense and lasts for a long time. Even though

GAD typically starts in adulthood, it can also affect teenagers. About 1% of younger and 3% of older teenagers may have GAD.

Interestingly, GAD is more commonly diagnosed in girls than in boys. It's also common for kids with GAD to experience other problems like depression simultaneously.

So, while some anxiety is normal in children, GAD is when it becomes solid, lasts a long time, and starts affecting their daily lives.

What causes generalized anxiety disorder in children?

Genetics and Anxiety: Studies involving families show that genetics can affect anxiety. Some kids might inherit a tendency to be anxious. It's not the only factor, however.

Environment Matters: Things in a child's life can also contribute to anxiety. For example, if a child goes through challenging or negative experiences or is around anxious people, it can make them more likely to be nervous.

Parents and Kids Influence Each Other: Anxiety can go both ways between parents and kids. If a child is anxious, it can affect how their parents behave, and how parents behave can also affect the child's anxiety.

Risk Factors: Some kids are more at risk of developing severe anxiety. These kids might struggle to pay attention, have a good relationship with others at school, and have parents who are very strict or discipline them a lot.

In simple terms, anxiety can be influenced by a mix of things, including our genes, what happens to us, and how we interact with our family and environment. Some kids are more likely to develop intense anxiety, especially if they have certain risk factors.

Treatment

CBT for Anxiety in Kids

First Choice: CBT (Cognitive-Behavioral Therapy) is usually the first choice for helping kids with anxiety. It's a talk therapy that teaches them how to manage their stress.

Working Together: The child and their parents must work with the therapist. Parents can learn how to support their child during therapy, and this teamwork is crucial.

Homework: Sometimes, kids have "homework" from therapy. This can be things like practicing relaxation exercises or changing how they think about their worries.

CBT Techniques: CBT uses relaxation exercises (to calm the body), changing how they think about their worries, and problem-solving skills (to deal with problems).

Different Settings: CBT can happen one-on-one with a therapist, with the family, in a group, or even at school. It's flexible to fit the child's needs.

In simple terms, CBT is a helpful therapy for anxious kids. It involves working together and learning new ways to cope with anxiety and can be done in places like a therapist's office or school.

Psychotherapy used to treat GAD.

Relaxation Techniques:

For children with GAD, relaxation techniques are like mental exercises that help them calm down when anxious. These techniques include deep breathing, where they take slow, deep breaths to relax their body. They might also learn muscle relaxation, where they tense and then release different muscles to release tension. These exercises can be like tools in their "mental toolbox" when anxiety starts to creep in. It's a way to tell their body, "It's okay to relax."

Mindfulness:

Mindfulness is like training your mind to focus on the present moment. Children with GAD often worry about things that might happen in the future. Mindfulness helps them pay attention to what's happening right now. It might involve simple activities like focusing on their breath or paying close attention to the sensations in their body. It's a way to gently steer their thoughts away from worries and into the present.

Gradual Exposure:

Sometimes, kids with GAD have fears or worries about certain things or situations. Gradual exposure is a way to help them face these fears slowly, step by step. For example, if a child is very anxious about dogs, they might first look at pictures of dogs, then watchdogs from a

distance, and eventually, with the help of a therapist, meet a friendly dog. This gradual approach helps them get used to what they fear in a safe and controlled way. Over time, the anxiety becomes less intense because they learn that the feared situation isn't as scary as they thought.

These techniques are like tools that therapists use to help kids with GAD learn to manage their anxiety, stay calm, and face their fears in a way that doesn't overwhelm them. It's all about helping them feel more in control and less anxious.

Separation Anxiety Disorder

Imagine feeling overwhelming fear and distress whenever you're apart from your loved ones, like your parents or caregivers. This is a daily reality for children with Separation Anxiety Disorder (SAD). SAD is not just about the usual worries children have when they leave home; it's an

intense and often disruptive anxiety levels can make everyday activities like attending school or staying at a friend's house daunting.

Common normal fears

Birth to 6 months   Loss of physical support, Loud noises, Large rapidly approaching objects 7–12 months   Strangers

1–5 years Loud noises, Storms, Animals, The dark, Separation from parents 3–5 years Monsters, Ghosts

6–12 years Bodily injury/sickness, Burglars, being sent to the principal Punishment, Natural disasters, Failure/rejection

12–18 years Tests in school, Low social competence, social evaluation, social embarrassment, psychological abnormality

How common is SAD?

Separation Anxiety Disorder, or SAD, affects about 3% to 5% of young people. It's more common in children than in teenagers. Interestingly, recent studies have shown that girls experience it more often than boys, although older studies didn't find this difference. Also, if

someone in your family has or has SAD, you might be more likely to experience it. Essentially, SAD can run in families. It's a condition where kids or teens worry a lot when they're separated from their loved ones, like parents, and it can make daily life more challenging for them.

What causes SAD?

Family and Genetic Factors: SAD tends to run in families, suggesting there could be a

genetic part. If someone in your family has SAD, you might also be more likely to get it. But it's not just about genes; it's also about how you're raised and what you learn from your family.

Developmental Theories: Some experts think that SAD might start when kids are very young and are trying to figure out how safe they are when they're away from their parents. It's normal for little kids to feel unsure when their mom or dad isn't around. But for some kids, this uncertainty continues as they grow up and can turn into SAD.

Behavioral Theories: This idea is about how our behavior and feelings are connected. SAD could be because of something called "conditioned fear," which means that you learn to be afraid of being apart from your loved ones, and this fear sticks around because it gets reinforced, like when you cry and your parents come back to comfort you.

Biological Theories: These theories focus on how our bodies and brains work. Some parts of our brain can handle fear and stress; if they don't work quite right, it might make SAD more likely. Also, if your parents or other family members have mood or anxiety problems, it might increase your chances of having SAD.

Temperamental Factors: This one is about your natural personality. Some kids are naturally more cautious and shyer when they face new or unfamiliar situations. If you're like this, it might increase your risk of developing SAD.

Parenting Styles: How your parents raise you can also play a role. For instance, if your parents are very controlling or don't give you much freedom, it might make you more anxious.

Remember, these are just different ideas, and SAD is likely caused by a mix of these factors working together. Researchers are still trying to understand it better.

How SAD is treated

Psychoeducation means teaching the child and their parents about SAD, helping them understand what's happening.

Collaboration with the Primary Care Provider: The doctor who cares for the child's overall health is involved in the treatment process.

School Consultation: If the child misses school because of SAD, working with the school to find solutions and get the child back to classes is essential.

Cognitive-Behavioral Therapy (CBT): This talk therapy helps children learn to manage their fears and worries. It can involve various techniques like relaxation exercises and changing negative thought patterns.

Family Therapy: Sometimes, SAD can affect the whole family. Family therapy can help everyone understand and cope with the condition.

Medication: Sometimes, a doctor might prescribe medication, like antidepressants. This is usually considered when other treatments aren't enough or when the anxiety is severe.

Returning to School: If the child is missing school, the goal is to help them return to school as soon as possible. The family and the school must work together to make this happen.

Sleep Issues: If SAD is causing sleep problems or the child is afraid to sleep alone, behavioral techniques can create a calming bedtime routine and help the child feel safe sleeping independently.

Parental Support: If a parent is also struggling with anxiety or mood issues, they might need treatment, including therapy or medication.

Transition Planning: Sometimes, the child might need to move from one level of care to another, like outpatient treatment to a day program. This transition should be planned carefully.

All these treatments aim to help the child feel more comfortable when separated from their parents and get back to their regular activities, especially school. Remember, treatment choice depends on the child's unique situation and what works best for them.

Social Anxiety Disorder

Picture a scenario where everyday social interactions, like meeting new people, speaking in front of the class, or joining group activities, want to face a relentless storm of anxiety. These situations can be incredibly distressing for children with Social Anxiety Disorder (SAD), affecting their self-esteem, relationships, and overall well-being.

How common is social anxiety disorder?

"Many kids have fears, like being scared of heights or spiders, but not all get help from doctors or therapists because parents and teachers don't always send them for treatment.

Around 5% of all kids and 16% of teenagers have these fears, which we call 'specific phobias.' Girls and younger kids tend to have them more often, although everyone is equally scared of needles.

Another kind of fear is called 'social anxiety disorder.' It's when kids fear being judged or embarrassed in front of others. This affects about 2% to 5% of kids, but some studies say it might be as high as 9% in teenagers and young adults. About 16% of the general population might have experienced it over time.

Usually, kids who get treatment for these fears are more anxious and might have other issues too."

What causes social anxiety disorder?

Kids can develop anxiety for different reasons. Some might be because of their genes or how they're naturally inclined to react to things. The environment they grow up in also plays a significant role. This includes their relationships with their parents, upbringing, how they get
along with friends, and if they go through challenging or stressful experiences. It's not just one thing, but a mix of everything working together.

How to identify a child with social anxiety disorder

When doctors want to understand if a child has a phobia or social anxiety, they usually talk to the child and sometimes the parents. Younger kids might be unable to explain it well, so they might show it through crying, upset, or clinging to someone. Older kids might quietly avoid what they're scared of or be irritable. The doctor asks questions to determine what the child fears, when it started, how they act when they're afraid, and if there are any reasons why they might not want to get better. Sometimes, they use questionnaires or tests to help measure how bad the anxiety is. It's essential to ensure it's not something else causing these feelings, like other mental health issues or learning problems.

How to overcome social anxiety disorder

Therapists often use different methods to help children with their fears. The best one is called cognitive-behavioral therapy (CBT). It's good at helping kids with phobias. CBT can also help with other fears kids might have. To do this, the therapist looks at the child's skills and teaches them new ones if needed. They also work with the family and school to stop things that might worsen the fear.

For specific fears, CBT methods that were made for grown-ups, like systematic desensitization and exposure therapy, can be used for kids, too. But they change them to fit the child's age and how they think. These methods might include slowly facing what they're afraid of in real life,
telling stories about it, showing them how others handle it, and using rewards and other tricks to help them get over their fear.

CBT involves three main parts:
Learning about what's going on in their head (psychoeducation).
Gradually facing situations that scare them (exposure therapy).

Learning how to be better in social situations (social skills).

There are guides and worksheets to practice things like talking to new people and how to act in social situations.

CBT also includes tricks like changing their thoughts (cognitive restructuring) to feel

better in scary situations. It's like turning their negative thoughts into positive ones. This helps them feel more confident and able to handle social situations.

Obsessive-Compulsive Disorder

Obsessive-Compulsive Disorder, or OCD, isn't just something that affects adults. It can also

affect kids. OCD is like having a bully in your brain. It makes you have unwanted thoughts that

bother you a lot and makes you do things repeatedly to push those thoughts to disappear. In this chat, we'll talk about OCD, how it

can show up in children, and what can be done to help.

How common is OCD among children?

OCD is a problem that's difficult to spot, especially in kids. It makes people have strange and upsetting thoughts that they can't control, and they do certain things repeatedly to make these thoughts disappear. This happens more than you might think, but many kids keep it a secret because they're embarrassed. It's estimated that OCD affects about 1% to 2% of children and teenagers, which means it's more common than you might realize. Sometimes, young kids also have habits like needing everything right or worrying about germs, but that's normal. OCD often starts in childhood, usually preadolescence, and sometimes it can come back in early adulthood. Boys often get it a bit earlier than girls, but it's about the same for both by the time they become teenagers. The excellent news is that OCD in kids tends to get better over time than when it starts in adulthood.

What causes OCD?

The exact cause of OCD (obsessive-compulsive disorder) in children isn't fully understood, but it's believed to result from a combination of factors:

Brain Chemistry: There might be differences in how certain chemicals in the brain, like serotonin, work in children with OCD. These chemicals help transmit signals between nerve cells and are linked to mood and behavior.

Genetics: OCD can sometimes run in families, suggesting a genetic component. If someone in the family has OCD, there may be a higher risk for other family members.

Stress and Trauma: Stressful life events, like family problems, illness, or significant life changes, can sometimes trigger or worsen OCD symptoms in children.

Infection and Autoimmune Factors: In some cases, streptococcal infections (such as strep throat) may be associated with the sudden onset of OCD symptoms, known as Pediatric. Autoimmune Neuropsychiatric Disorders Associated with Streptococcal Infections (PANDAS). However, this is not a common cause of OCD.

Environmental Factors: Certain environmental factors could play a role in the development of OCD, but more research is needed to understand these connections better.

Remember, it's usually a combination of these factors rather than a single cause contributing to OCD in children.

How OCD Present in children

Obsessive-Compulsive Disorder (OCD) in children is identified by the presence of obsessions
and compulsions that are distressing and time-consuming. Here are some standard features of OCD in a child:

Obsessions are painful and invasive ideas, images, or urges that a youngster has regularly. Children frequently develop obsessions, such as worries about contamination, hurting others, or things being out of order. These ideas significantly increased my fear.

Compulsions: Compulsions are recurrent actions or thoughts that a youngster feels compelled to conduct to ease the suffering brought on by their obsessions. These actions might be overt. (noticeable) or covert (rituals of the mind). Examples include washing your hands, checking your locks, counting, or silently repeating things.

Time-Consuming: Obsessions and compulsions can take up much of the child's time. They may spend hours daily performing rituals or trying to resist their obsessions.

Interference: OCD can interfere with the child's daily life, including school, social activities, and family life. It may affect their ability to concentrate and perform well in school.

Anxiety and Distress: Children with OCD often experience high levels of stress and distress due to their obsessions and compulsions. They may recognize that their thoughts and behaviors are irrational but still find them challenging to control.

Resistance: Children with OCD usually don't want to have these obsessions or perform these compulsions, but they feel driven to do so to relieve their anxiety.

Avoidance: Some children may try to avoid situations or places that trigger their obsessions, which can limit their activities and social interactions.

Many kids with OCD know that their obsessions and compulsions are excessive or unreasonable, yet they are powerless to control them.

Many kids with OCD often have recurring thoughts that bother them a lot. These thoughts can be about things like dirt, germs, inappropriate sexual reviews, or feeling like they're doing something wrong. To cope with these thoughts, they might do things like washing their hands
over and over, repeating actions, checking things repeatedly, or arranging stuff in a particular order.

How to treat a child with OCD

Cognitive-behavioral therapy (CBT) for OCD in children is a structured, practical, first-line approach to help them manage their obsessive thoughts and compulsive behaviors.

Exposure and Response Prevention (ERP): ERP is a central component of CBT for OCD. It involves deliberately exposing the child to situations that trigger their obsessions while preventing them from engaging in compulsive behaviors. For example, suppose a child is obsessed with germs and compulsively washes their hands. In that case, the therapist might gradually expose them to a slightly dirty object and help them resist the urge to wash their hands immediately.
Over time, this helps the child realize that their fears are unfounded, and they can resist the compulsions.

Cognitive Restructuring: This part of CBT helps the child identify and challenge irrational thoughts related to their obsessions. They learn to replace these negative thoughts with more realistic and less distressing ones.

Mindfulness and Relaxation Techniques: Children with OCD often experience high anxiety levels. Mindfulness and relaxation exercises can help them manage their anxiety and reduce the need for compulsive behaviors.

Homework: The child is given "homework" assignments to practice what they've learned during therapy sessions. This helps reinforce the skills they're developing and allows them to generalize these skills to real-life situations.

Gradual Progress: CBT for OCD is a gradual process. The therapist works with the child to
create a hierarchy of fears, starting with less distressing situations and gradually moving to more challenging ones.

Pharmacological treatments

Medication should be considered when OCD symptoms are severe, in the presence of comorbid disorder or family dysfunction, when the patient or family resists engaging in CBT, or when a skilled CBT clinician is unavailable.

Medication can be valuable in treating Obsessive-Compulsive Disorder (OCD), especially in certain situations. Here are some key factors to consider when deciding if medication should be included in the treatment plan for OCD:

Severity of Symptoms: Medication is often considered when OCD symptoms are severe and significantly interfere with a child's daily life, such as their school performance, relationships, or overall functioning.

Comorbid Conditions: If a child with OCD has other mental health conditions, such as depression or anxiety disorders, medication may be recommended to address these comorbidities simultaneously.

Family Dysfunction: In cases where family dynamics contribute to or exacerbate the child's OCD symptoms, medication can help reduce anxiety levels, making it easier for the family to engage in therapy and implement effective strategies.

Resistance to CBT: Some children and their families may resist engaging in cognitive-behavioral therapy (CBT), the primary psychotherapy for OCD. Medication can be considered when there's significant resistance to CBT.

Limited Access to Skilled CBT: In some areas, finding a therapist experienced in CBT for OCD can be challenging. If access to a skilled CBT clinician is limited, medication may be a reasonable alternative or complement to treatment.

Previous Treatment Outcomes: Medication can be explored as an adjunct to therapy if the child has previously tried CBT without success or has relapsed after initially responding to treatment.

Preference and Comfort: The child's and family's preferences and comfort with medication should also be considered. Some families may be more open to medicines as part of the treatment plan, while others may prefer to start with therapy alone.

Risks and Benefits: Parents and healthcare providers must discuss the potential risks and benefits of medication. This includes considering side effects and how they might impact the child's quality of life.

Monitoring and Adjustments: Medication for OCD should always be closely monitored by a healthcare provider. The child's response to the medication, any side effects, and changes in symptoms should be carefully tracked, and adjustments made as necessary.

It's important to note that medication should not be the sole treatment for OCD in children.
It should be used with evidence-based psychotherapy like
cognitive-behavioral therapy (CBT), particularly exposure and response prevention (ERP). The combination of CBT and medication is highly effective in managing OCD symptoms.

The decision to consider medication in the treatment of OCD should be made collaboratively between the child's parents, healthcare providers, and mental health professionals. The goal is to create a comprehensive treatment plan tailored to the child's needs and circumstances.

Relapse Prevention: Once the child has progressed, they learn strategies to prevent relapses and maintain their gains.

Role of parents

OCD is a Real Medical Condition: OCD does not result from bad parenting or something a child is doing on purpose. It's a legitimate medical condition that affects the brain's functioning.

Understanding Obsessions and Compulsions: OCD is characterized by obsessions (repeated, intrusive, and distressing thoughts) and compulsions (repetitive behaviors or mental acts performed to reduce anxiety). These obsessions and compulsions can be very disturbing for the child.

Early Intervention is Crucial: Identifying and addressing OCD early is essential. The earlier the treatment begins, the better the outcomes tend to be.

Treatment is Available: Effective treatments for OCD are available, including cognitive-behavioral therapy (CBT) and, in some cases, medication. Parents should work closely with mental health professionals to determine the best treatment plan for their child.

CBT and Exposure Therapy: Cognitive-behavioral therapy, particularly exposure and response prevention (ERP), is often the first-line treatment for OCD in children. In ERP, the child gradually faces their fears and learns not to engage in compulsions. Parents may need to be involved in supporting their children during these exposures.

Medication Can Help: In some cases, medication, typically selective serotonin reuptake inhibitors (SSRIs), may be prescribed to manage OCD symptoms. Parents should discuss the benefits and potential side effects of medication with their child's doctor.

Be Patient: Recovery from OCD is a gradual process, and there may be setbacks. Parents should be patient and supportive during their child's treatment journey.

Avoidance Makes OCD Worse: Avoiding situations that trigger OCD symptoms can worsen the condition. Encouraging the child to confront their fears, with the guidance of a therapist, is an essential part of treatment.

Positive Reinforcement: Providing praise and rewards for facing fears and resisting compulsions can be highly effective in motivating a child during treatment.

Open Communication: Encourage your child to talk openly about their OCD symptoms and feelings. A supportive and non-judgmental environment can make a significant difference.

Advocacy: Advocate for your child at school and in social settings. Educate teachers, counselors, and other caregivers about your child's condition and the necessary accommodations.

Self-Care: Remember to take care of yourself as a parent.

Supporting a child with OCD can be emotionally taxing, so seek support from other parents, support groups, or mental health professionals when needed.

Overall, parents should approach OCD with empathy, understanding, and a commitment to helping their child access the appropriate treatment and support they need to manage their condition effectively.

Chapter 5: Mood Disorders

Disruptive Mood Dysregulation Disorder (DMDD)

Disruptive Mood Dysregulation Disorder (DMDD) was introduced to give a proper label to a group of kids and teens who were previously labeled with bipolar disorder. DMDD came about from studying a group of kids with severe irritability and restlessness that resembled some aspects of mania, but not exactly.

Unlike classic bipolar disorder, these kids didn't experience distinct mood episodes. They had other conditions like ADHD, defiance, and anxiety. They also had a different brain profile. As they grew up, they were more likely to develop depression and anxiety, not bipolar disorder.

To diagnose DMDD, a child must show a whole year of being constantly irritable and having severe outbursts that don't match the situation. These outbursts must happen often and not just at home. The child's behavior affects their life at home, school, and with friends. DMDD can't be diagnosed if a child has certain other conditions. There's still a lot to learn about DMDD and how it's different from other disorders, so more research is needed.

HOW COMMON IS DMDD

Disruptive Mood Dysregulation Disorder (DMDD) is a newly diagnosed mental illness, and its reported prevalence rates vary depending on the population studied. Here's what we know in simple terms:

Community Samples: In studies involving kids from the general population, DMDD is less common. It affects about 1% of children aged 9 to 17 years.

Preschool Children: The rate is higher in very young children (ages 2 to 5 years), with about 3.3% meeting the criteria for DMDD.

Clinic Settings: In clinical settings like outpatient clinics, DMDD rates are significantly higher. For instance, in one study, 26% of children aged 6 to 12 met the DMDD criteria when seeking help. Over two years, this number increased to 40%.

Comorbidities: DMDD often occurs alongside other conditions like Oppositional Defiant
Disorder (ODD), Conduct Disorder, and depressive disorders. For example, in one study, 92% of children with DMDD also had symptoms of ODD.

Overlapping with ODD: There's a significant overlap between DMDD and ODD, which has led to some questioning whether DMDD should be considered a separate diagnosis or just a specifier of ODD.

In a nutshell, DMDD is more prevalent in clinical settings, often coexisting with other disorders like ODD. Its validity as a distinct diagnosis is still discussed among experts.

Causes

As DMDD is a new diagnosis, little is known about its etiology. A family history of bipolar disorder may increase the risk of DMDD.

Challenges

Young adults who used to meet the criteria for DMDD when they were kids have more anxiety, depression, and other mental health issues than adults. They also have worse physical health, less money, and more legal problems, and they don't do as well overall compared to those who didn't have DMDD as kids.

Treatment

There aren't clear treatment rules for DMDD yet. However, some early studies show that stimulant medications and a medicine called risperidone might help. Valproate has shown promise in reducing aggression in kids with ADHD, defiance, and conduct issues.

In a new study, stimulants helped kids with both ADHD and

DMDD. They had better attention, fewer depressive feelings, and less defiance. But even with treatment, many kids still face challenges.

Anger Management Techniques:

Children with DMDD often struggle with intense outbursts of anger and irritability. Anger management techniques help them learn how to handle and express their anger better. These techniques might include things like:

Deep Breathing: Teaching the child to take deep breaths when they start to feel angry can help calm their emotions.

Counting to Ten: Encouraging them to count slowly to ten before reacting when they're upset, giving them time to think.

Identifying Triggers: Helping them recognize what makes them angry so they can work on those situations.

Positive Self-Talk: Teach them to replace negative thoughts with positive ones so they don't get overwhelmed by anger.

Collaborative Problem-Solving with Families:

DMDD doesn't just affect the child; it can also significantly impact the family.

Collaborative problem-solving involves working closely with the child's family to find solutions. This might include:

Family Therapy: Having therapy sessions with the whole family to improve communication and understanding.

Setting Clear Expectations: Creating clear rules and expectations at home to reduce conflicts.

Positive Reinforcement: Encourage and reward positive behavior to reinforce good actions.

Stress Reduction for Parents: Helping parents manage their stress because this can affect how they respond to their child's behavior.

These techniques create a supportive and structured environment for the child with DMDD. It helps them learn how to manage their anger and behavior while involving the family to ensure a more harmonious home life.

Chronic major depressive disorder and persistent depressive disorder

Major Depressive Disorder in Children:

Major Depressive Disorder (MDD), also known as clinical depression, affects children similarly to adults but with unique characteristics. Kids with MDD often experience persistent sadness, irritability, or hopelessness. They may lose interest in activities they once enjoyed, have changes in appetite or sleep patterns, and lack energy. Physical complaints like headaches or stomachaches might be expected.

Other signs include difficulty concentrating, feeling guilty or worthless, and thoughts of death or suicide. Children with MDD might withdraw from friends and family, and their school performance might decline. It's important to note that MDD can manifest as physical symptoms rather than just emotional ones.

Persistent Depressive Disorder (PDD) in Children:

Persistent Depressive Disorder, also called Dysthymia, is a long-lasting form of depression. Children with PDD experience a consistently low or sad mood for at least a year. This chronic sadness might come and go, but it doesn't go away entirely for an extended period.

Kids with PDD may have the same symptoms as MDD but on a milder level. They might feel down than usual, have low self-esteem, and lack interest in everyday activities. PDD can affect their social interactions, school performance, and overall well-being.

Genetic factors, life stressors, and brain chemistry can cause MDD and PDD in children. Early identification and proper treatment are essential to help children manage these conditions and lead fulfilling lives.

How common is this?

The rate of major depression is around 1%-3% in younger children and 3%-9% in teenagers.

These numbers can change based on who is being studied, how depression is defined, and how it's measured. In a study, about 20%-25% of teens experienced at least one episode of major depression by late adolescence. Another study found that about 3% had a condition called

dysthymic disorder. Many more young people have signs of feeling down, even if they don't have full-blown depression. Before puberty, boys and girls have similar rates of depression. But as they become teenagers, girls are more likely to experience it, just like adults.

Causes

What causes mood disorders in kids is like what causes them in adults. If a parent is depressed, it can be passed down genetically or because the child learns from them. The risk can also increase if parents are distant or not emotionally available. Bad experiences like abuse and neglect can be a reason, especially for young children.

Challenges

Childhood mood disorders are severe and can even lead to fatal outcomes. In a study, 4% of children with major depression had died by suicide. In another study, around 8% of those with teenage-onset depression had taken their own lives. The risk of suicide is higher if there's a history of previous suicide attempts, substance abuse, easy access to dangerous things (like guns), impulsive behavior, conduct issues, family history of suicide attempts, or abuse.

The earlier depression starts, the longer and more severe it tends to be, often running in families. Over the past few decades, major depression has started at a younger age. In one study, the average length of a depressive episode in kids was nine months. Dysthymia, another kind of

depression, lasted about four years. Many times, dysthymia turned into major depression. Kids who recover often face a high risk of more episodes and other issues. Children with early-onset depression are more likely to develop bipolar disorder later. For teens with significant depression, signs like sudden symptom onset, slow movement, psychotic features, or a family history of bipolar disorder can predict the development of bipolar disorder.

Treatment

When kids show risky behavior or think about suicide, they need careful supervision from parents and mental health professionals. Sometimes, kids might need to stay in a hospital if they're very sad or having dangerous thoughts and don't get better with regular visits to the doctor.

For kids with mild to moderate depression, around 60% get better with supportive care. But when depression starts early in life, it can significantly impact how they grow up. Long-term help is often necessary. Even after they feel better, therapy might be needed to work on coping skills, thinking, and good relationships with others.

Family involvement is significant for kids, even more than for adults. Learning about the condition (psychoeducation) and knowing how to prevent it from coming back (relapse prevention) can be helpful for both kids and families.

Therapy usually comes first for depression without severe problems. Medication can be added if it doesn't help in a few weeks. For more severe depression, medication might be the starting point. Two medicines, fluoxetine (for ages eight and up) and escitalopram (for ages 12 and up), are approved by the FDA for treating childhood major depression.

For kids whose depression does not improve with one medicine, adding therapy to a different drug seems to work better than switching medications. In severe cases where other treatments have not worked, electroconvulsive therapy might be considered.

Kids with seasonal affective disorder might benefit from bright light therapy in the mornings.

Bipolar Disorder in Children

Bipolar Disorder in children, sometimes called Pediatric Bipolar Disorder, is a psychiatric condition that brings extreme mood alterations. These mood swings can be intense, ranging from high-energy episodes, excitement, and impulsivity (mania or hypomania) to periods of deep sadness and hopelessness (depression).

What makes pediatric bipolar disorder unique is that these mood changes can happen more rapidly and intensely than in adults with bipolar disorder. Children with this condition may also have other challenges, like difficulty in school or relationships.

Diagnosing and treating bipolar disorder in children can be complex, but early intervention and proper management can help kids lead fulfilling lives despite this condition's challenges. Understanding the signs, symptoms, and available treatments is essential for parents, caregivers, and healthcare professionals to provide the best support for children with bipolar disorder.

How common

Bipolar disorder in children is quite rare. It's uncommon to see the extreme highs and lows associated with this condition in young kids. However, as teenagers age, the chances of experiencing these mood swings become more like what adults with bipolar disorder go through.

In a study of high school students, about 1% had experienced bipolar disorder. Another 5.7% had symptoms like bipolar disorder but not as intense.

Interestingly, 45% of children and teens initially diagnosed with a milder form of bipolar disorder developed the more severe types of bipolar disorder over five years. Having a family history of bipolar disorder was a vital sign that this might happen.

About 20% of all people with bipolar disorder have their first episode during their teenage years. So, while it's not common in kids, it becomes more noticeable as they age.

What causes bipolar disorder in children?

Sometimes, it's not easy for adults to notice when kids have mania or hypomania (extreme energy and excitement). Kids might do risky things, act overly excited, or show much interest in grown-up topics like sex. Remember that just because a child works this way doesn't mean they've been abused. It could be a sign of mania.

Kids with mania might also believe they're unique or essential, which is different from regular bragging or make-believe. They might not want to sleep much, but it's not the same as having trouble sleeping because they resist bedtime or use substances.

Family history and how things have been over time can help doctors determine if a child might have bipolar disorder. Kids who develop bipolar disorder when they're young tend to

They have a more challenging time than those who get it as adults. They often have other issues like anxiety, behavior problems (ADHD or defiance), or substance problems.

Research suggests that anxiety disorders might be one of the first signs in people who later develop bipolar disorder. So, if a child has anxiety issues and a family history of bipolar disorder, doctors might pay extra attention.

Treatment

Treating bipolar disorder in young people can be tricky because it's hard to do scientific studies on them. We can't always use what works for adults because it doesn't always work for kids.

In addition to medicine, some therapies can help, especially for teenagers. These include Family-Focused Treatment for Adolescents, family therapy, and cognitive-behavioral therapy for both the child and the family. These therapies can be added to medication to improve treatment results.

Mood Stabilization Strategies and care

Children with Bipolar Disorder often experience extreme mood swings between mania (high energy, impulsivity, and irritability) and depression (low mood, sadness, and lack of energy). Mood stabilization strategies aim to balance these mood swings and help children maintain a more stable emotional state. These strategies might include:

Therapy: Psychotherapy, especially Cognitive-Behavioral Therapy (CBT), can help children learn to manage their emotions and develop coping skills.

Routine: Establishing a daily routine can provide structure and predictability, which can help stabilize moods.

Healthy Lifestyle: Encouraging regular exercise, a balanced diet, and proper sleep can positively impact mood stability.

Safety Planning and Crisis Management:

Safety planning is crucial when dealing with Bipolar Disorder, especially if a child experiences severe mood episodes or thoughts of self-harm or suicide. Here's how it works:

Identifying Triggers: Recognizing what situations or events might trigger severe mood swings or crisis moments.

Emergency Contacts: Having a list of emergency contacts, including therapists, doctors, and trusted individuals, to reach out to during a crisis.

Crisis Response: Knowing what to do in a crisis, such as following a specific plan, staying with the child, or seeking immediate medical help.

Safety Measures: Taking precautions to ensure the child's safety during extreme mood episodes, like removing any potential hazards.

Safety planning and crisis management are essential to ensure the child's well-being during
severe mood swings, and they involve careful preparation, communication, and quick response to keep the child safe.

These strategies aim to provide support and stability for children with Bipolar Disorder, helping them manage their mood swings and stay safe during challenging moments.

Chapter 6: SLEEP-WAKE DISORDERS

Sleep disorders in children are quite common, with 25% of all kids experiencing them at some point. These disorders involve issues with the quality, timing, and amount of sleep, which

can lead to daytime distress and problems functioning. Some common sleep problems in children and teenagers include sleep talking, nightmares, waking up during the night, difficulty falling asleep, bedwetting, teeth grinding, rocking in sleep, restless legs syndrome, and nightmares.

In a survey among adolescents, about 10% reported having experienced difficulties with falling asleep, staying asleep, or feeling excessively sleepy during the day at some point in their lives.

Children with chronic medical conditions, neurodevelopmental disorders, or psychiatric disorders are at a higher risk of experiencing sleep problems. For example, 30% to 80% of children with intellectual disabilities and 50% to 70% of children with autism spectrum disorder (ASD) have associated sleep issues.

Sleep problems can also be linked to mood and anxiety disorders, so assessing a child's sleep is essential when evaluating their mental health. The DSM-5 (Diagnostic and Statistical Manual of

Mental Disorders, Fifth Edition) provides guidelines for categorizing and diagnosing sleep disorders, helping healthcare professionals better understand and address these issues in children.

Insomnia in Children

Causes and Treatment

Insomnia in children is persistent difficulties falling or staying asleep, leading to impaired daytime functioning. It's more common in younger children and often involves bedtime resistance and nighttime awakenings. Some infants may experience irregular sleep patterns during their first year.

Various factors can contribute to insomnia in infants and toddlers, including perinatal complications, separation anxiety, and disruptions in parent-child interactions. In preschoolers, daytime napping schedules can affect nighttime sleep. Chronic insomnia is more prevalent in children with psychiatric disorders, such as ADHD, oppositional defiant disorder, or separation anxiety disorder. It can also be a symptom of mood disorders, autism spectrum disorder (ASD), or schizophrenia. Additionally, substance use, including caffeine or medications, can disrupt sleep.

When addressing insomnia in young children, it's crucial to

eliminate factors hindering sleep and establish bedtime routines. Behavior modification techniques can reduce nighttime awakenings and reinforce positive sleep habits. Hypnosis or relaxation techniques may benefit older children and adolescents.

Behavior therapy can help break the association between bedtime anxiety and sleep difficulties in adolescents with insomnia. Improving sleep hygiene involves using the bed only for sleeping, following a regular sleep schedule, avoiding daytime naps, and removing electronic devices from the bedroom. Cognitive-behavioral therapy is effective for older children and teens.

While hypnotic medications are not recommended for chronic use in children, melatonin, a hormone that assists with circadian regulation, may be helpful for short-term use in some cases, with minimal adverse effects. Currently, there are no FDA-approved medications specifically for pediatric insomnia treatment. A consistent approach among family members is essential for successful management.

Narcolepsy

Understanding and Managing

Narcolepsy is a rare sleep disorder characterized by several symptoms, but not all children or adolescents with narcolepsy experience it all. The main symptoms are daytime sleepiness, cataplexy (sudden muscle weakness or loss of muscle tone), hypnagogic hallucinations (vivid dream-like experiences), and sleep paralysis (temporary inability to move or speak when falling asleep or waking up). For a diagnosis, these symptoms must be accompanied by specific test results, such as cerebrospinal fluid (CSF) hypocretin deficiency, rapid eye movement (REM) sleep latency in nocturnal polysomnography (PSG), or shortened mean sleep latency in multiple sleep latency tests (MSLT) with at least two sleep-onset REM periods.

Narcolepsy typically begins in late adolescence or early adulthood and can significantly disrupt daily life, including school performance and relationships. The diagnosis is often challenging due to its rarity, and other potential causes of daytime sleepiness must be considered first.

Treatment involves educating the patient and their family about narcolepsy, maintaining a regular sleep schedule with planned naps, and using medications to manage specific symptoms. Stimulant drugs like methylphenidate and dextroamphetamine can help reduce sleep attacks, especially during school hours. Modafinil is a non-stimulant medication that promotes wakefulness and is FDA-approved for narcolepsy. Sodium oxybate is effective for excessive daytime sleepiness in narcolepsy. Medications like tricyclic antidepressants and selective serotonin reuptake inhibitors may be used to manage cataplexy, sleep paralysis, and hypnagogic hallucinations.

Early diagnosis and appropriate management can significantly improve the quality of life for individuals with narcolepsy.

Obstructive Sleep Apnea (OSA): Understanding and Managing

Obstructive sleep apnea (OSA) is a common sleep disorder characterized by episodes where breathing temporarily stops or is partially blocked, leading to lower oxygen levels in the blood. Signs of OSA in children include frequent snoring, observed instances of interrupted breathing or gasping for air during sleep, restless sleep, and sweating at night. It's estimated that OSA affects about 1% to 4% of children, with higher rates among those with certain medical conditions or
genetic syndromes.

OSA occurs when the upper airway becomes blocked, often due to structural or neurological factors. When this happens, the child's body works harder to breathe, sometimes leading to partial awakenings. Several factors can contribute to OSA, including obesity, enlarged tonsils and adenoids, asthma that worsens at night, floppy airway tissues, facial or jaw abnormalities, neuromuscular conditions, Down syndrome, and hypothyroidism.

Diagnosing OSA typically requires a sleep study called polysomnography (PSG). Children with OSA may experience health complications, including problems with the heart and growth, like high blood pressure and failure to thrive. Additionally, OSA can affect a child's behavior and school performance, causing developmental delays, irritability, aggression, distractibility, inattentiveness, and hyperactivity.

The primary treatment for OSA is often surgical, involving the removal of enlarged tonsils and adenoids, which is successful in most cases. Continuous positive airway pressure (CPAP) therapy, which consists of wearing a mask that helps keep the airway open during sleep, is an

alternative for children who haven't responded to surgery or are not suitable candidates for it. Early diagnosis and proper management can significantly improve the quality of life for children with OSA.

Understanding Restless Legs Syndrome (RLS)

Causes and treatment.

RLS is a condition where people have a solid impulse to move their legs, frequently accompanied by painful leg sensations. The need is typically eased by moving one's legs during rest when it is worse in the evening or at night. It is vital to remember that youngsters may not always refer to these feelings as "urges." Between 2% and 7% of the population are thought to be affected by RLS; it is more common in women and becomes more likely as people age. While RLS usually manifests in adolescence, some persons with the condition recall having symptoms as early as late childhood or adolescence.

The causes of RLS can vary. Iron deficiency is one potential factor, as RLS is more common in individuals with this deficiency.

There is also a vital genetic component, with higher rates among people of European descent than African or Asian descent. RLS has been associated with disruptions in the central dopaminergic system.

Treatment for RLS involves both behavioral and pharmacological approaches. Behavioral strategies include maintaining a regular sleep schedule, avoiding sleep deprivation, reducing caffeine intake, refraining from tobacco and alcohol use, and avoiding stimulating activities close to bedtime. Iron supplementation may be recommended for children with iron deficiency.

Dopaminergic medications are safe and well-tolerated in children. Additionally, drugs like gabapentin have shown effectiveness in treating pediatric RLS. Other medications, such as benzodiazepines, α-agonists, and carbamazepine, can also be considered for managing RLS in children.

Understanding Nightmare Disorder

Nightmare disorder involves experiencing frightening dreams, which is expected during REM (rapid eye movement) sleep, especially in the latter part of the night. When a child wakes up from a nightmare, they usually become alert and can recall the dream. While some children may go back to sleep quickly, others may find it challenging and request to sleep with their parents. The frequency of nightmares can vary throughout a child's development.

In kids aged 3 to 5 years, between 10% and 50% may have recurring nightmares that disturb their parents. Typically, these symptoms start during preschool and become less frequent as the child ages. In some cases, nightmare disorder may persist into adulthood.

Nightmare disorder in children is not consistently linked to any specific psychiatric conditions.

Factors such as stress, sleep deprivation, fatigue, and changes in the sleep environment can

contribute to an increase in nightmares. Medications may also sometimes lead to more frequent nightmares. The best approach for managing nightmare disorder is often reassurance. Children should not be pressured to describe their nightmares but should be allowed to talk about their fears. Normalizing sleep schedules and increasing sleep time, especially if the child is sleep-deprived, can be helpful. For children and adolescents with more persistent issues, anxiety reduction techniques like relaxation, imagery with systematic desensitization, and dream

reorganization may be beneficial. If nightmares are a symptom of post-traumatic stress disorder or another underlying condition, addressing the primary cause is essential.

Chapter 7: Disruptive Behavior Disorders

Oppositional Defiant Disorder

Most people affected by oppositional defiant disorder (ODD) are children and adolescents. ODD is a complex and frequently misunderstood behavioral illness. A pattern of rebellious, disobedient, and angry behavior toward caregivers such as parents, teachers, or other authoritative figures is what defines it. Children with ODD frequently display a recurrent pattern of antagonistic, combative, and defiant behaviors that go beyond ordinary oppositional or rebellious conduct in children.

Due to the many arguments, disciplinary problems, and strained relationships that ODD can cause, it can be challenging for the child and their family to go about their everyday lives. Parents, educators, and mental health professionals must comprehend ODD, its symptoms, and its causes to support and intervene on behalf of children with this illness.

How common is ODD?

The varying criteria used to diagnose Oppositional Defiant Disorder (ODD) have made it challenging to determine its exact prevalence. According to the DSM-5, prevalence estimates range widely, from 1% to 11%, with an average estimate of around 3.3%. ODD affects boys slightly more than girls, with similar or slightly higher rates.

ODD is frequently observed in clinical settings, such as psychiatric clinics and special education classrooms. It often co-occurs with attention-deficit/hyperactivity disorder (ADHD).

What causes ODD?

Various psychosocial models have been proposed to understand the causes of Oppositional Defiant Disorder (ODD). They all share a common idea: there is a pattern of negative interaction between parents and children, which leads to inconsistent discipline, a lack of structure, and
difficulties in setting limits. This, in turn, reinforces oppositional behavior in the child.

Parents of children with ODD often experience marital problems, although it's challenging to determine whether these problems contribute to the disorder or result from raising a difficult child. Genetic, neurobiological, and temperamental factors may also play a role. ODD and a
problematic temperament in children can have significant similarities, making it difficult to distinguish between them. Additionally, environmental factors like poverty, family

dysfunction, child abuse, and parental mental health issues have been linked to an increased risk of ODD.

How to identify a child with ODD

Identifying a child with Oppositional Defiant Disorder (ODD) can be challenging, but several signs and behaviors may suggest ODD's presence. These include:

Frequent and Persistent Anger: Children with ODD often exhibit intense and frequent anger beyond typical temper tantrums and may become easily annoyed or lose their temper regularly.

Frequent Arguments: ODD children tend to argue with adults and authority figures, such as parents, teachers, and caregivers, more often than their peers.

Defiance and Refusal to Comply: They often refuse to comply with rules, requests, or instructions, even when they understand them. This defiance can be directed at parents, teachers, or other authority figures.

Blame-Shifting: Children with ODD may frequently blame others for their mistakes or misbehavior and refuse to take responsibility for their actions.

Vindictiveness: ODD children may be spiteful or vindictive, seeking revenge or intentionally trying to annoy others.

Frequent Loss of Temper: They may have frequent and severe temper outbursts disproportionate to the situation.

Argumentative Behavior: These children often argue with adults, particularly authority figures.

Difficulty with Peer Relationships: ODD can impact a child's ability to form and maintain friendships, as they may have trouble cooperating and having good relationships with their peers.

Defiance at School: ODD can also manifest in the school setting, with children exhibiting disruptive or defiant behavior toward teachers and classmates.

It's important to note that while these behaviors can indicate ODD, they may also occur in response to other issues or developmental stages. A qualified mental health professional, such as a child psychologist or psychiatrist, should conduct a comprehensive evaluation to make an
accurate diagnosis and develop an appropriate treatment plan if ODD is suspected.

The treatment of Oppositional Defiant Disorder (ODD)

Oppositional Defiant Disorder (ODD) treatment typically involves a multimodal approach, addressing various aspects of the child's behavior and environment. Here are some.

Common treatment modalities for ODD:

Parent Management Training (PMT): PMT is a core component of ODD treatment. It helps parents develop practical parenting skills to manage their child's behavior. This includes strategies for setting clear expectations, using consistent consequences, and improving communication.

Individual Therapy: Individual therapy for the child with ODD can help them understand and manage their emotions and behaviors. Cognitive-behavioral therapy (CBT) techniques may teach coping skills and problem-solving strategies.

Family Therapy: Family therapy involves working with the entire family to improve communication, reduce conflicts, and build stronger relationships. It can help parents and siblings better understand and support the child with ODD.

Behavioral Interventions: These interventions focus on modifying specific behaviors associated with ODD. Behavioral strategies include reinforcement and consequences to encourage positive behaviors and discourage negative ones.

Social Skills Training: Children with ODD often struggle with social interactions. Social skills training can teach them appropriate ways to interact with peers and adults.

Medication: In some cases, when ODD is accompanied by other conditions such as ADHD or mood disorders, medication may be prescribed to address those coexisting issues. Drugs should be considered carefully and are usually used in conjunction with psychotherapy.

School-Based Interventions: Collaborating with teachers and school staff is essential. Special education services, individualized education plans (IEPs), and 504 programs can provide additional support at school.

Parent Support and Education: Providing parents with support and education about ODD can help them better manage their child's behavior and reduce stress within the family.

Skill-Building Programs: Programs that focus on developing the child's social and emotional skills, problem-solving abilities, and anger management can be beneficial.

Community Resources: Accessing community resources, such as support groups for parents or extracurricular activities for the child, can help build a strong support network.

Treatment plans are individualized based on the child's unique needs and the severity of their symptoms. Early intervention and a consistent, structured approach to treatment can lead to positive outcomes for children with ODD. Parents and caregivers need to work
closely with mental health professionals to develop and implement an effective treatment plan.

Conduct Disorder

Conduct Disorder (CD) in children is a complex and severe behavioral disorder characterized by a persistent pattern of behaviors that violate the fundamental rights of others or societal norms and rules. These behaviors are often aggressive, antisocial, and disruptive, causing significant impairment in a child's daily life and functioning. CD is typically diagnosed in childhood or adolescence, but its effects can extend into adulthood if left untreated.

Key features and behaviors associated with Conduct Disorder include:

Aggression: Children with CD often engage in physical aggression toward people, animals, or property. This may consist of bullying, fights, and causing harm to others.

Destruction of Property: They frequently engage in vandalism or intentional destruction of property without regard for the consequences.

Deceitfulness: Children with CD may lie, steal, or engage in dishonesty, such as shoplifting, forgery, or breaking.

Violation of Rules: They consistently disregard rules, defy authority figures, and refuse to comply with established guidelines at home, in school, or in the community.

Cruelty to Others: Some children with CD exhibit cruel behavior toward people or animals, including physical harm, bullying, and intimidation.

Lack of Empathy: There is a notable absence of empathy or remorse for the harm caused to others. Children with CD may not understand or care about the feelings of others.

Frequent Truancy: They may skip school without valid reasons, leading to academic problems.

Substance Abuse: Adolescents with CD are at a higher risk of engaging in substance abuse and experimenting with drugs or alcohol.

It's important to note that occasional disobedience or rule-breaking is common among children and adolescents. However, CD is diagnosed when these behaviors become pervasive, persistent, and severe, causing significant impairment in multiple areas of a child's life.

How standard is CD

The DSM-5, a manual doctors use to understand mental health conditions, tells us that Conduct Disorder (CD) varies in how common it is among kids and teenagers in the United States. It can affect anywhere from 2% to over 10% of young people. Even though more girls are experiencing CD nowadays, it's still more common in boys. For every girl with a CD, about 3 to 4 boys have it.

Boys tend to commit more violent crimes related to CD compared to girls, with an 8 to 1

difference. But when we look at what kids report about their behavior, the gender gap becomes smaller. In those cases, it's more like two boys with a CD for every one girl. This difference might have to do with how society thinks about gender, race, and how much money families have. These factors can influence whether someone is recognized as having a CD.

Also, it's worth noting that Conduct Disorder is something that doctors often see in young people who visit outpatient psychiatric services, clinics, or programs for helping with mental health.

Causes for developing CD.

A combination of factors can influence the development of Conduct Disorder (CD) in children and adolescents, and it's often not just one single cause. Here are some of the critical factors that can contribute to the development of CD:

Biological Factors: Genetics can play a role in CD. A child may be at a higher risk if there is a family history of CD or other behavioral disorders.

Brain Structure and Function: Differences in brain structure and function, particularly in impulse control and decision-making, can be associated with CD.

Environmental Factors: Adverse environments, such as exposure to violence, abuse, neglect, or trauma during childhood, can significantly increase the risk of developing CD.

Parenting Style: Inconsistent or harsh parenting, lack of supervision, and poor parent-child attachment can contribute to CD. Children who haven't learned appropriate behavior from their parents are more likely to develop CD.

Peer Influence: Associating with peers who engage in delinquent or antisocial behaviors can also contribute to the development of CD. Peer pressure to engage in rule-breaking activities can be a powerful influence.

Socioeconomic Factors: Growing up in communities with high crime rates, limited access to quality education, and economic hardship can increase the risk of CD.

Substance Abuse: Substance abuse, especially at an early age, can contribute to developing and worsening CD symptoms.

Psychological Factors: Certain psychological factors, like a lack of empathy or guilt, can also play a role in CD.

It's important to remember that not all children exposed to these risk factors will develop CD. Many children face challenges but do not develop this disorder. The interplay of these factors is complex, and early intervention and support can be effective in helping children manage and
overcome CD.

Treatment and management options for a child with CD

Treating and managing Conduct Disorder (CD) in children typically involves a combination of therapeutic approaches and interventions. Working closely with mental health

professionals to develop an individualized treatment plan is essential. Here are some standard treatment and management options:

Behavioral Interventions: These interventions focus on changing the child's behavior and teaching them more appropriate ways to interact with others. They may include:

Parent-Child Interaction Therapy (PCIT): A therapist coaches' parents on effective discipline and communication techniques.

Parent Management Training (PMT): Parents learn how to reinforce positive behaviors and set clear consequences for negative behaviors.

Functional Family Therapy (FFT): The whole family participates in therapy to improve communication and resolve conflicts.

Individual Therapy: In one-on-one therapy sessions, children can explore the underlying causes of their behavior and learn strategies for managing anger, frustration, and impulsivity.

Medication: Medication may be considered if the child has comorbid conditions like ADHD, depression, or anxiety. Drugs like stimulants or mood stabilizers may be prescribed, but they are typically used in conjunction with therapy.

School-Based Interventions: Collaboration with the child's school is essential. Behavioral intervention plans, special education services, and counseling can help address conduct problems in an educational setting.

Social Skills Training: Teaching the child appropriate social skills, problem-solving, and conflict resolution can improve their interactions with peers and adults.

Parent Education and Training: Parents play a crucial role in managing CD. Learning effective parenting techniques, communication skills, and strategies for setting and enforcing boundaries is essential.

Family Therapy: Family therapy can address family dynamics and conflicts that may contribute to the child's behavior problems. It can also improve communication and strengthen family bonds.

Community Programs: Involvement in community-based programs, such as mentoring, youth groups, or sports teams, can provide positive outlets for the child's energy and help them develop social skills.

Crisis Intervention: In some cases, crisis intervention may be necessary to ensure the child's safety and that of others. This may involve hospitalization or temporary removal from the home.

Long-Term Follow-Up: CD can persist into adolescence and adulthood. Long-term monitoring and support may be necessary to prevent further problems and legal issues.

It's essential to tailor the treatment plan to the child's specific needs and involve a team of professionals, including therapists, counselors, educators, and, when necessary, psychiatrists.

Early intervention and consistent, structured support can significantly improve the child's chances of managing and overcoming CD.

Chapter 8: Neurodevelopmental Disorders

Autism Spectrum Disorder

Autism Spectrum Disorder (ASD) is a developmental condition that can impact how children think, feel, and interact with the world around them. It's like having a unique way of seeing and experiencing things. Kids with ASD might struggle to understand social cues and emotions, making communication and building relationships tricky. They might have specific interests or routines they enjoy and find comfort in.

Some children with ASD may have challenges with language, such as difficulty starting conversations or understanding jokes. Repetitive behaviors, like repeating words or doing the same actions repeatedly, are also common.

It's important to remember that every child with ASD is different, and their strengths and difficulties can vary. Early identification, intervention, patience, and support from parents, caregivers, and educators can make a big difference in helping kids with ASD learn and grow.

How common is ASD (epidemiology)

Prevalence of ASD: This means how common Autism Spectrum Disorder (ASD) is in the population. The most recent data from the CDC says that for every 1,000 children who are eight years old, about 14 to 15 have ASD. So, it's not extremely common, but it's not super rare either.

Increase in Prevalence: Over the years, the number of kids diagnosed with ASD has increased. Between 2002 and 2010, it increased by 123%, but it leveled off between 2010 and 2012. This increase is mainly because doctors are better at recognizing ASD, and the rules

for diagnosing it has become broader.

Boys vs. Girls: Boys are more likely to have ASD than girls. For every four boys with ASD, there's about one girl with it. Scientists are still figuring out why this is.

Racial Differences: White children are more likely to be diagnosed with ASD than Hispanic or Black children. This might be because some families from different backgrounds face challenges getting their kids assessed and treated for ASD.

So, in simple terms, ASD is not super rare, but it's not super common either. More kids are being diagnosed with it because we're getting better at spotting it, but there are still some differences in who gets diagnosed based on their gender and race.

What causes ASD?

Genetics and Autism: Autism Spectrum Disorder (ASD) can run in families. If a child has ASD, their siblings also have a 4.5% chance of having it. Twins can help us understand this better. If one identical twin has ASD, there's a higher chance (60% to 90%) that the other twin will have it too. But it's not always the case, which means that other things, like early environmental factors, might also play a role.

No Blame on Parents: It's important to know that autism is not caused by how parents raise their children or any social or emotional factors. It's mostly linked to genetics and some environmental factors.

Specific Genetic Causes: In some cases (about 15%), doctors can identify a particular genetic reason for autism. This usually happens when a child with autism has severe developmental delays, intellectual disabilities, or physical differences. Some known genetic causes include
fragile X syndrome and specific chromosomal issues.

Other Risk Factors: Some things that might increase the chance of a child having autism include older parents (both moms and dads), having a sibling with autism, being born prematurely, or having pregnancies close together.

Vaccines and Autism: Many studies have looked at vaccines, like the MMR vaccine, but have found no link between vaccines and autism. So, getting vaccinated to prevent diseases is safe and doesn't cause autism.

In simple terms, autism often runs in families, but it's not anyone's fault, especially not the parents. Sometimes, a specific genetic cause can be found, but usually, it's a mix of genes and other factors. Vaccines do not cause autism; they are safe and essential for health.

Diagnosing Autism Spectrum

Diagnosing Autism Spectrum Disorder (ASD) involves looking at a child's behavior, communication skills, and development. Doctors and specialists often use a combination of observations, interviews with parents, and standardized tests to make an assessment.

Early signs of ASD can become noticeable as young as 18 months old. These signs may include:

Social Challenges: Children might need to avoid eye contact, not respond to their name being called, or need help understanding and using gestures like waving or pointing.

Communication Differences: Kids may not start talking as early as their peers or have trouble conversing. They could only repeat phrases after fully understanding their meaning.

Repetitive Behaviors: Children might engage in repetitive movements, like rocking or hand-flapping, or become intensely focused on specific interests or objects.

Rigidity with Routine: A strong desire for routines and difficulty with plan changes or transitions can be a sign.

Sensory Sensitivities: Children might be overly sensitive to lights, sounds, textures, or tastes.

It's important to remember that having some of these traits doesn't necessarily mean a child has ASD. However, if you notice a consistent pattern of these behaviors and if they interfere with a child's daily life and learning, it's a good idea to seek professional evaluation. Early intervention services can provide support and strategies to help children develop essential skills.

Strategies for managing ASD.

Supporting a child with Autism Spectrum Disorder (ASD) involves understanding their strengths and challenges and tailoring interventions accordingly. Here are ways to offer support and some behavioral interventions that can be helpful:

Support Strategies:

Structured Routine: Establish a consistent daily routine, as predictability can comfort children with ASD.

Clear Communication: Use simple language, visual aids, and gestures to help convey information effectively.

Positive Reinforcement: Praise and reward desired behaviors to motivate the child to repeat them.

Sensory-Friendly Environment: Create a calm space with sensory accommodations to help the child manage sensory sensitivities.

Social Skills Training: Teach and practice social interactions through role-playing and guided activities, like taking turns and making eye contact.

Emotional Understanding: Use visuals or stories to help the child recognize and label different emotions.

Individualized Education: Collaborate with teachers to create a personalized education plan that addresses the child's unique needs.

Behavioral Interventions:

Applied Behavior Analysis (ABA): A structured approach that breaks down skills into smaller steps and uses positive reinforcement to encourage desired behaviors.

Picture Exchange Communication System (PECS): A visual communication system using pictures to help children express their needs and desires.

Social Stories: Short stories that explain social situations and expected behaviors, helping children understand and navigate social interactions.

Discrete Trial Training (DTT): Using repetitive teaching methods to help children learn specific skills, often used in ABA therapy.

Token Economy: Using tokens or points as rewards for desired behaviors, which can be exchanged for preferred activities or items.

Visual Schedules: Visual schedules or charts outline daily routines and activities, providing structure and predictability.

Functional Communication Training (FCT): Teaching alternative ways to communicate effectively, such as using words or gestures, to replace challenging behaviors.

Working with professionals, such as behavior therapists, speech-language pathologists, and occupational therapists, is essential to determine the most appropriate interventions for the child's needs. Additionally, the child's caregivers and educators should be involved in creating a consistent and supportive environment across different settings.

Attention-Deficit/Hyperactivity Disorder

Attention-Deficit/Hyperactivity Disorder (ADHD) in children is a neurodevelopmental condition that significantly affects their ability to focus, control impulses, and regulate their energy levels. It's a common pediatric disorder impacting children's academic performance, social interactions, and overall well-being. Children with ADHD often exhibit various behaviors, including difficulty staying attentive in tasks, acting impulsively without considering consequences, and being overly active or restless.

ADHD is more than just a passing phase of childhood; it can persist into adolescence and adulthood if left untreated. The challenges posed by ADHD can extend beyond the individual child, affecting family dynamics and interactions with peers and educators. However, with

appropriate understanding, early identification, and a comprehensive approach to treatment and support, ADHD children can thrive and harness their unique strengths. This involves medical interventions, tailored behavioral strategies, educational accommodations, and cultivating self-awareness and coping skills.

How common is ADHD?

The number of children having ADHD varies because it depends on how we measure it and where we look. The official estimate in the DSM-5 is about 5% of school-age kids. However, when we look at different studies, we can see a wide range. In some studies, 17% of boys and 8% of girls in elementary school are said to have ADHD. In adolescence, it's about 11% of boys and 6% of girls. So, it's more common than you might think.

Boys vs. Girls: It's important to know that ADHD is seen more often in boys than in girls. In clinical settings, there are about nine boys with ADHD for every one girl. But in community surveys, it's closer to 2 to 3 boys for every one girl. Girls with ADHD are more likely to have the type where they struggle with paying attention but aren't hyperactive or impulsive. They're also more likely to have other issues like anxiety or depression.

ADHD Worldwide: ADHD isn't just an American thing. It's found in many countries around the world. However, how we diagnose and treat it can vary depending on location. In the U.S., because kids are expected to go to school until they're 18, we often catch ADHD because it affects how they do in school. They might notice it less in other countries because kids aren't in school as long.

Gender and Diagnosis: One important thing to remember is that sometimes, girls with ADHD might not get identified or treated as often as boys with ADHD. However, the symptoms and how they affect their lives can be very similar.

So, in simple terms, ADHD is quite common and found worldwide. Boys are more often diagnosed, but girls can have it, too. How we see and treat ADHD can differ depending on where we live and what people expect from kids in school.

What causes ADHD?

The causes of ADHD are a bit like a puzzle with missing pieces, and scientists are still figuring it out. Here's what we know in simple terms:

Genes: One big piece of the puzzle is genetics. ADHD tends to run in families, so if someone in your family has it, you might be more likely to have it, too.

Brain Differences: Another piece is about how the brain works. In people with ADHD, certain parts of the brain that help with focus and self-control might not work as well as they should.

Pregnancy and Birth: Things that happen before a baby is born or during birth can also play a role. For example, if a mom smoked or drank during pregnancy, it might increase the chances of her child having ADHD.

Chemicals in the Brain: Tiny chemicals called neurotransmitters help the brain communicate. Some research suggests that in people with ADHD, these chemicals might not work perfectly.

Environment: Sometimes, things in a person's background, like lead exposure or certain pesticides, could be factors. But this is still being studied.

Sugar and Food: People used to think that overeating sugar or certain foods caused ADHD, but there's no substantial proof.

Remember, it's like a giant puzzle, and each person's dilemma might differ. Researchers are working hard to understand all the pieces and how they fit together.

Identifying Attention-Deficit/Hyperactivity Disorder (ADHD)

Identifying Attention-Deficit/Hyperactivity Disorder (ADHD) in preschool-age children requires a keen understanding of typical developmental milestones and the early signs that may indicate the presence of the condition. Both parents and preschool teachers play a crucial role in recognizing potential ADHD-related behaviors. Here's how they can identify the state:

Parents:

Observation: Parents should observe their child's behavior in different settings, not just at home. Notice if certain behaviors are consistently present and causing challenges.

Comparison: Compare the child's behavior with that of their peers. If there are significant differences in attention, impulsivity, or activity levels, it might be worth exploring further.

Developmental Milestones: Be aware of typical developmental milestones for preschoolers, such as attention span, self-control, and appropriate social interactions.

Consultation: If concerns arise, consult a pediatrician or mental health professional. They can provide guidance and conduct a more thorough assessment.

Preschool Teachers:

Behavior Patterns: Pay attention to behavior patterns that deviate from typical preschooler
behavior, such as difficulty following instructions or staying engaged in activities.

Comparisons: Compare the child's behavior with that of their classmates. Persistent and notable differences warrant closer attention.

Inattentiveness: Observe if a child consistently struggles to focus on tasks, has trouble listening during group activities, or becomes easily distracted.

Impulsivity: Note if a child frequently interrupts others, has trouble waiting their turn, or seems unaware of personal space boundaries.

Hyperactivity: Be attentive to excessive restlessness, fidgeting, difficulty remaining seated, and being unusually energetic.

Communication: Maintain open communication with parents. If there are consistent concerns about the child's behavior, discuss your observations with the parents and encourage them to seek professional evaluation.

Documentation: Keep records of specific behaviors, instances, and patterns you observe. This documentation can be helpful when discussing concerns with parents or professionals.

It's important to remember that ADHD diagnosis is a complex process that involves thorough assessment by qualified healthcare professionals. Parents and teachers should collaborate and share observations, which can contribute to a comprehensive understanding of the child's
behavior and needs. Early identification and appropriate interventions can make a significant difference in supporting children with ADHD to succeed in preschool and beyond.

Behavioral Strategies for ADHD children:

Clear Instructions: Provide simple instructions and break tasks into smaller steps to make them more manageable.

Positive Reinforcement: Use praise, rewards, and small incentives to encourage and reinforce desired behaviors.

Routine and Structure: Establish consistent habits for daily activities, which can provide predictability and help manage impulsivity.

Visual Aids: Use visible schedules, charts, and reminders to help children understand expectations and transitions.

Task Organization: Teach organizational skills like using color-coded folders, labels, and checklists to help keep track of assignments and belongings.

Time Management: Introduce techniques like timers and alarms to help children manage time effectively.

Social Skills Training: Teach appropriate social interactions, sharing, and taking turns through role-playing and guided activities.

Cognitive Interventions for ADHD:

Cognitive Behavioral Therapy (CBT): Help children recognize and challenge negative thought patterns, develop coping strategies, and enhance impulse control.

Mindfulness and Self-Regulation: Teach mindfulness techniques to increase awareness of thoughts and emotions, fostering better self-regulation.

Problem-Solving Skills: Help children develop strategies for decision-making, planning, and considering consequences before acting.

Executive Function Training: Focus on improving executive functions like working memory, planning, and cognitive flexibility through targeted exercises.

Role of Parents:

Education: Learn about ADHD, its symptoms, and available strategies for managing it.

Consistency: Establish consistent routines, rules, and expectations at home.

Positive Reinforcement: Use praise and rewards to reinforce positive behaviors.

Communication: Maintain open contact with teachers and mental health professionals to monitor progress.

Supportive Environment: Create an organized, low-distraction home environment.

Encourage Physical Activity: Promote regular physical activity to help manage excess energy.

Role of Preschool Teachers:

Observation: Observe and document behavior patterns to provide valuable information for assessment.

Structure: Create a structured classroom environment with clear routines and expectations.

Individualized Approach: Tailor strategies to each child's needs and strengths.

Positive Reinforcement: Praise and acknowledge good behavior to boost self-esteem. **Collaboration**: Communicate observations and concerns with parents and professionals. **Patience and Empathy**: Understand that children. You may need extra support and patience.

Collaboration between parents, preschool teachers, and mental health professionals is essential for successfully managing ADHD in children. By working together and using a

combination of behavioral strategies and cognitive interventions, they can develop coping skills, improve self-regulation, and succeed in both academic and social settings.

When considering medication options for children with Attention-Deficit/Hyperactivity Disorder (ADHD), it's essential to prioritize safety and effectiveness. Here are some medication options and critical considerations specifically for children:

Important Considerations for Children:

Expert Consultation: The decision to use medication should involve a child psychiatrist or pediatrician with expertise in ADHD treatment.

Comprehensive Assessment: Thorough evaluation includes medical history, family history, physical exam, and assessment of any coexisting conditions.

Lowest Effective Dose: Medication should be started at the lowest effective dose and adjusted carefully under medical supervision.

Monitoring: Regular check-ups are necessary to assess medication effectiveness, side effects, and any needed adjustments.

Side Effects: Parents should be aware of potential side effects, such as appetite changes, sleep disturbances, and mood swings.

Long-Term Considerations: The child's growth, development, and potential impact on school performance should be carefully monitored.

A trial period of medication, usually a few weeks, helps determine its effectiveness and tolerability.

Combined Approach: Medication is often more effective with behavioral therapies, educational support, and lifestyle adjustments.

Communication: Open communication between parents, teachers, and healthcare providers is crucial for monitoring progress and addressing concerns.

Counseling and Education: Both parents and children should be educated about ADHD, its treatment options, and strategies for managing symptoms.

Remember, every child is unique, and the choice to use medication is personal. The goal is to enhance the child's functioning and quality of life while minimizing potential risks. A collaborative approach involving healthcare professionals, parents, and teachers can lead to the best outcomes for children with ADHD.

Intellectual Disabilities [intellectual developmental mental disorder]

Intellectual Disabilities [intellectual developmental mental disorder] in children, also called intellectual developmental disorders, are conditions characterized by limitations in intellectual functioning and adaptive behavior. These limitations manifest during the developmental period and significantly impact the child's ability to learn, communicate, solve problems, and perform everyday tasks.

How common are intellectual disabilities?

Prevalence: This means how often something occurs. In the United States, the occurrence of Intellectual Disabilities (ID) can vary, but on average, it affects 1% to 3% of the population. So, it's not super common, but it's not extremely rare either.

Gender Difference: ID is more common in males. This means boys are about 30% more likely to have ID than girls. However, this difference becomes smaller when we look at more severe forms of ID.

So, in simpler terms, ID is a condition affecting how people think and learn. It's uncommon but often seen in boys, especially in milder forms. But remember, each person is unique, and ID can vary in severity.

What causes intellectual disabilities?

There are many reasons why someone might have intellectual disabilities. In about 30% of cases, we don't know the exact cause. However, some known factors that can increase the risk of intellectual disability include being born with low weight, being male, having mothers of specific ethnic backgrounds, having older mothers, having lower maternal education, having lower income, having multiple births (like twins), or being a second or later-born child.

Most Cases Linked to Social and Genetic Factors: Most cases of intellectual disability are thought to be a combination of genetic factors (things you inherit from your family) and social factors (like your environment and upbringing).

Severity Matters: When intellectual disability is more severe, it's less likely to be from unknown causes. In these cases, we can often identify a biomedical reason, which means a physical or genetic explanation.

Common Genetic Causes: Down syndrome is a well-known genetic cause of intellectual disability. It's usually due to a mistake in how a mother's cells divide. Fragile X syndrome is.
Another common genetic cause. It's linked to certain physical features and behavioral traits like hyperactivity and social anxiety.

Differences in Strengths and Weaknesses: People with these conditions may have unique strengths and weaknesses. For example, individuals with Down syndrome might be better at visual tasks but struggle with language. It's essential to understand and support these

differences.

So, in simpler terms, intellectual disabilities can have various causes, and sometimes, we don't know the exact reason. Genetic and social factors often play a role. Well-known conditions like Down syndrome and Fragile X syndrome can cause intellectual disabilities, each with its characteristics. People with these conditions have strengths and challenges; supporting and understanding them is essential.

How to diagnose intellectual disabilities

Parents might suspect their child has Intellectual Disabilities (ID) based on a combination of developmental milestones, behaviors, and observations. Remember that every child develops at their own pace, so it's essential to consult a healthcare professional for an accurate assessment. Here are some signs that might raise concerns:

Developmental Milestones:

Delays in Milestones: Noticeable delays in achieving developmental milestones like sitting up, crawling, walking, or talking.

Speech and Language: Severe speech delays or difficulty communicating and understanding language appropriate for their age.

Motor Skills: Struggles with fine and gross motor skills, such as holding a pencil, using utensils, or walking smoothly.

Behavioral Observations:

Limited Problem-Solving: Difficulty solving fundamental problems or completing simple tasks typical for their age.

Learning Challenges: Difficulty learning and retaining new information or needing help to catch up with peers academically.

Social Interaction: Challenges in social interactions, making friends, understanding social cues, or sharing interests.

Adaptive Behavior:

Self-Care Skills: Struggling with activities of daily living such as dressing, grooming, or feeding oneself independently.

Safety Awareness: Lack of understanding about basic safety precautions, like crossing the street or staying away from dangerous objects.

Other Considerations:

Regression: Loss of previously acquired skills or a noticeable deterioration in development.

Consistency: If these behaviors or delays are consistent over time and not simply a phase.

Comparison: Comparing the child's development to peers of the same age can help identify potential differences.

Parental Instinct: Sometimes, parents have an intuitive sense that their child's development is not progressing as expected.

Can Coexist with other neurodevelopmental disorders.

The prevalence of co-existing Attention-Deficit Hyperactivity Disorder (ADHD) among individuals with ID falls between 4% and 11%, resembling figures found in the general population. A noteworthy companion to ID is Autism Spectrum Disorder (ASD), with significant overlap. 30%-40% of those with ID also exhibit ASD, while conversely, 70% of individuals with ASD have ID.

Depression can emerge due to ID, stemming from added burdens, self-esteem challenges, and social stigmatization. It's also occasionally coincidental, with prevalence matching or surpassing the general population.

Around 25% of young individuals encounter notable anxiety symptoms within the realm of ID. Diagnoses encompass Generalized Anxiety Disorder (GAD), various phobias, panic disorders,

Posttraumatic Stress Disorder (PTSD) and Obsessive-Compulsive

Disorder (OCD).

If parents have concerns about their child's development or suspect Intellectual Disabilities, it's essential to take the following steps:

Consult a Professional: Schedule an appointment with a pediatrician or developmental specialist who can conduct a thorough evaluation.

Early Intervention: If concerns are validated, seek early intervention services, which can provide support and therapies tailored to the child's needs.

Observe and Document: Keep track of the child's behaviors, milestones, and any patterns of concern to share with healthcare professionals.

Seek Multiple Opinions: Don't hesitate to seek a second opinion if your concerns must be addressed adequately.

Remember that early identification and intervention can significantly impact a child's development and potential. It's always best to consult healthcare professionals for accurate assessments and guidance.

Specific Learning Disorders

Specific Learning Disorders (SLD) are neurodevelopmental conditions that affect the acquisition and use of academic skills. These disorders manifest as difficulties in reading, writing, mathematics, or a combination of these areas. Despite having average or above-average intelligence, individuals with SLD struggle to master specific skills related to language and numbers.

With impairment in reading, specify if deficits in [dyslexia]

Word reading accuracy.

Reading rate or fluency

Reading comprehension

With impairment in mathematics, specify if deficits in [dyscalculia]

Number sense

Memorization of arithmetic facts

Accurate or fluent calculation

Accurate math reasoning

With impairment in written expression, specify if deficits in [dysgraphia]

Spelling accuracy

Grammar and punctuation accuracy

Clarity or organization of written expression

What causes this?

Genetics plays a significant role in specific developmental disorders. Family histories often show increased occurrences of reading, speech, and language disorders among parents and siblings of affected children. However, the inheritance pattern needs to be more consistent. Twin studies indicate substantial genetic influence, with high concordance rates in identical twins (85%-70%) and

lower rates in non-identical twins (50%-45%).

Male prevalence is notable (at least 2:1). Developmental reading disorders can also relate to maternal smoking during pregnancy, low birth weight, and prenatal/perinatal factors, alongside genetic influences.

Challenges

Learning disorders often go unnoticed, presenting as school refusal, oppositional defiant
disorder, depression, or somatoform disorder. Children affected by these disorders might feel embarrassed by academic challenges, develop a dislike for school, and avoid schoolwork.
Diagnoses typically arise during grade school years. While milder cases can improve with ongoing support and practice, organization issues persist even after addressing fundamental skills. As individuals progress to higher education, struggles with foreign languages, writing, and reading might continue. Emotional and behavioral challenges often persist beyond

The initial developmental deficits. Learning disorders can lead to low

self-esteem, anxiety, and difficulties coping with frustration. Associated problems encompass truancy, delinquency, and school dropout. Links between learning disorders, ADHD, and heredity are notable. Complex interactions also exist with conduct disorder. Comorbid depression or anxiety disorders are common.

Treatment

Many specialists and teachers may work together to help when a child faces learning challenges and multiple difficulties. All these people need to talk to each other, especially when the child changes schools. A unique way to help kids is called "Response to Intervention" (RTI). It means giving extra help to struggling kids in school before saying they have a learning problem. The additional support and the way the child responds can help us understand and treat the issue.

The IDEA law says all kids with problems, like learning difficulties, have the right to get a good education that suits their needs. This might include special classes or help, depending on their struggle. Their plan for each child is called an "Individualized Education Plan" (IEP). Kids might get special tools like calculators, more time for tests, or help from a tutor.

Parents are critical in planning their child's education. Talking to a counselor might help parents understand how to be positive and supportive. Kids with these difficulties can still

achieve a lot, even if they learn a bit slower. Therapy can help kids feel better about themselves and handle anger or frustration. Sometimes, if there are other issues like ADHD, medication can help. But for learning problems specifically, medication doesn't usually help.

Chapter 9: Substance Use and Addictive Disorders

Substance use and addictive disorders in children are a growing concern today. These issues involve young individuals using various substances, such as drugs or alcohol, in a manner that can lead to addiction and significant health, social, and psychological problems. Understanding and addressing substance use and addiction in children is crucial for their well-being and the well-being of society. This introduction will overview the challenges and complexities associated with substance use and addictive

disorders in children, highlighting the importance of early intervention and support for affected youth.

Surveys done on substance use in the younger population.

Three national surveys tell us how many young people use drugs and alcohol. One called "Monitoring the Future" asks around 50,000 students in 8th, 10th, and 12th grades about their drug and alcohol use every year. However, the numbers might not be completely accurate because some of the heaviest drug users might not be in school or might not be there when the surveys are done.

Another survey is called the "National Survey on Drug Use and Health." The Substance Abuse and Mental Health Services Administration does it every year. This survey uses a computer-based questionnaire and tells us about drug and alcohol use in people 12 years and older.

The third survey is done by the Centers for Disease Control and Prevention every two years, called the "Youth Risk Behavior Surveillance System." This one focuses on behaviors that can hurt young people's health, like drug and alcohol use, risky sexual behaviors, and tobacco use.

How many children and teenagers are addicted to substances and addictive.

In 2015, a survey called "Monitoring the Future" discovered that fewer teenagers were smoking cigarettes and drinking alcohol compared to the previous year. However, the use of marijuana and e-cigarettes remained about the same. One concerning finding was that among 12th graders, more were using marijuana daily (6%) than tobacco. Also, fewer 12th graders thought marijuana was risky.

Another survey in 2015 called the "Youth Risk Behavior

Surveillance System" showed that
fewer young people were trying cigarettes and smoking them regularly. Alcohol use has also
decreased since 1991, but the rates were like those in 2013. Many high school students (45%) said they had tried electronic vapor products. Some students reported using prescription drugs that weren't prescribed to them (17%).

There are also new and unusual substances that some young people are using, like synthetic drugs and various herbs. These substances can be dangerous, and sometimes, they don't appear on regular drug tests. Some illegal drugs might even be mixed with deadly substances like fentanyl, which can be sold as heroin.

Adverse psychological issues with the use of substances

Teenagers who struggle with substance use often have multiple substance use problems. They can also have other issues like ADHD (Attention-Deficit/Hyperactivity Disorder), ODD (Oppositional Defiant Disorder), CD (Conduct Disorder), depression, anxiety disorders, PTSD
(Post-Traumatic Stress Disorder), psychosis, and specific learning disorders. Any mental health problem can be connected to substance use, either causing it, resulting from it, or happening simultaneously. Some teens might have these mental health

problems before they start using substances, while others might develop them because of the drugs they use.

A study that followed teenagers over time found that significant depression and heavy smoking made each other more likely in the future. This connection doesn't seem to be because they share the same risk factors. When ADHD is present, especially along with ODD or CD, it can lead to starting substance abuse at an early age.

Risk factors associated with severe substance abuse in adolescence.

Early Childhood Trauma: Experiencing trauma, such as physical or sexual abuse, at a young age can increase the risk of turning to substances to cope with the pain and emotional distress.

Rebelliousness: Teens who are consistently defiant and resistant to authority figures are likelier to engage in substance abuse.

Aggression: Those with aggressive behaviors are at a higher risk of using drugs and alcohol to express or manage their anger.

Impulsivity: Teens who act without thinking about the consequences of their actions may be more prone to experimentation with drugs and alcohol.

Low Self-esteem: Adolescents may turn to substances to feel better about themselves or to fit in with specific peer groups.

Elementary School Underachievement: Struggling academically in elementary school can be a red flag, as it may lead to feelings of failure and a greater likelihood of engaging in substance abuse.

Failure to Value Education: Teens who do not see the value in education may be more susceptible to risky behaviors, including substance abuse.

Absence of Strong Religious Convictions: Religious beliefs can serve as

protective factors against substance abuse for some teens. Lacking these convictions may increase vulnerability.

Experimentation with Drugs at a Young Age: Trying drugs or alcohol before age 15 is a significant risk factor for developing more severe substance abuse problems later.

Peer Influence: Having friends who engage in problematic behaviors, including drug use, can strongly influence a teenager's substance use.

Alienation from Parents: Feeling disconnected or distant from parents can contribute to substance abuse, as teens may seek connection or escape through drugs and alcohol.

Lack of Positive Family Dynamics: Families that lack precise discipline, positive reinforcement, and healthy relationships may contribute to an environment where substance abuse is more likely.

Family History of Substance Abuse: A family history of substance abuse can increase genetic and environmental susceptibility to addiction.

It's important to recognize these risk factors early and provide appropriate support and intervention to reduce the likelihood of severe adolescent substance abuse. Early prevention and intervention programs can address these risk factors and promote healthier choices among teenagers.

How substance use starts and where it leads the child into

Substance use can become a significant concern during adolescence. It often starts with trying things like cigarettes or alcohol and then progresses to more severe substances. This progression can lead to problems in various areas of life.

Gateway Progression: Many adolescents start with cigarettes or alcohol and then move on to more complex substances. For example, they might go from trying cigarettes to drinking beer or wine, then hard liquor, and eventually to marijuana and other illegal drugs. This progression often follows a predictable pattern.

Changing Landscape: With the legalization of marijuana for medical and recreational use in some places, there's concern that marijuana is becoming a gateway drug for some teens. This means they may start with marijuana and skip the earlier stages of tobacco and alcohol use.

Potency Concerns: The marijuana available today is much stronger than before. This increased potency can have more significant effects on young users.

Continued Use: Usually, substances from each stage are continued into the next, leading to a pattern of abusing multiple drugs. Inhalant abuse is an exception, as many children may start with inhalants but then move on to other drugs.

Progression Risks: While many young people experiment with substances, only a fraction go on to regular use, and even fewer become dependent. Predicting who will progress to more severe substance use is challenging, but starting early and rushing increases the risk of serious problems.

Developmental Impact: Substance use during childhood and adolescence can interfere with the development of cognitive, social, and physical abilities. Missing critical experiences can lead to difficulties in the future.

Morbidity and Mortality: Substance use among youth can lead to a range of problems, including suicidal thoughts and behaviors, accidental overdoses, dangerous behavior while intoxicated (Like car accidents), and even homicide related to drug involvement. Chronic marijuana use can result in apathy and hinder academic and social development.

Health Risks: There's growing concern about the potential risks of heavy marijuana use on
cognitive function, motivation, and even the development of psychotic disorders in adolescents.

HIV and Other Risks: Injection drug use is a significant way HIV spreads among adolescents. It also puts them at risk for hepatitis. Substance use can lead to risky sexual behavior, which increases the chances of exposure to HIV and other sexually transmitted diseases.

Pregnancy Risks: Adolescent girls who use drugs may become pregnant, potentially putting their unborn child at risk for drug-related harm or HIV infection.

Substance use during adolescence can have far-reaching consequences, impacting various aspects of a young person's life and increasing the risk of severe health and social problems. Addressing substance use issues early is essential to minimize these risks and provide appropriate support and intervention.

How to overcome

The main goal of treating substance use in children and adolescents is to help them achieve and maintain abstinence from drugs or alcohol. Here's a summary of the critical aspects of treatment:

Abstinence Focus: The primary objective is to help young individuals stop using substances. Medical detoxification, which removes drugs or alcohol from the body, is rarely needed for adolescents.

Developmentally Appropriate Approaches: Treatment programs are tailored to the specific needs of young people, considering their developmental stage.

Group Therapy: Many treatment programs involve group therapy, where adolescents with

similar substance use issues come together to discuss their challenges and support each other in recovery.

12-Step Programs: Participation in self-help programs like Alcoholics Anonymous (AA) and Narcotics Anonymous (NA) is encouraged. These programs emphasize recovery as an ongoing process rather than a quick fix.

Addressing Denial and Peer Influence: Conventional individual psychotherapy may be less effective due to denial, lack of motivation, and peer pressure to use drugs. Therefore, alternative approaches are used.

Limited Use of Medications: Medications for substance use disorders are rarely used in adolescents. Treatment success is often associated with the patient's motivation, cooperation, willingness to undergo urine testing, and remaining in treatment for an extended period.

Sometimes, medications can help by addressing other psychiatric disorders, reducing withdrawal symptoms, or supporting abstinence.

Legal Interventions: In some cases, legal interventions and sanctions may be necessary to encourage compliance with treatment.

Therapeutic Techniques: Treatment approaches often include motivational interviewing, teaching social skills, strategies for problem-solving, coping, and relapse prevention. Structured and supervised recreational activities with drug-free peers are encouraged.

Addressing Comorbid Disorders: If there are other psychiatric disorders or learning disorders present, they need to be assessed and treated. However, a valid assessment may be challenging without a period of abstinence.

Educational and Vocational Support: Academic deficits should be addressed, and vocational testing and training may benefit older adolescents who may not return to traditional schooling.

Family Involvement: Family therapy approaches are practical.

These therapies focus on improving parent-youth relationships, addressing interaction patterns, and providing behavior management skills training for parents. Some models also involve peers, teachers, and other aspects of the youth's social environment. Family Therapy: Involving the family is a vital part of treatment. The goals include educating parents about substance abuse, improving parenting skills, and enhancing communication within the family. Parents may also need help with substance use or other mental health issues.

Short-Term Hospitalization: This is typically reserved for cases with acute medical issues, overdose, intoxication, or severe psychiatric conditions that pose immediate harm. The patient and family should be actively involved in group treatment and drug education.

Residential Treatment: This is used for severe, complex, or stubborn cases, especially when a parent is also dealing with substance abuse. It can last from 1 to 12 months.

Long-Term Continuation: After initial treatment, ongoing support is crucial. This can be in the form of outpatient programs, day treatment programs, or halfway houses. Active participation in groups like Alcoholics Anonymous (AA) or Narcotics Anonymous (NA) is often necessary.

Age-Appropriate Groups: Adolescents tend to do better in treatment groups with other adolescents rather than mixed with adults.

Positive Outcomes: Effective treatment leads to reduced substance abuse, better school performance, and fewer behavioral and psychological problems.

It's important to understand that relapses, or moments when a young person returns to using drugs, can happen during treatment. These should be seen as expected challenges, not disasters that mean the treatment has failed.

To help prevent relapses, treatment may include strategies to deal with situations where drug use is likely. This can help reduce the number and seriousness of relapses. Additionally, regular urine tests can support the goal of staying drug-free.

Chapter10: Exploring the Future of Child Psychiatry

Advances and Ongoing Research

Introduction

Child psychiatry is a rapidly evolving field dedicated to understanding and addressing mental health issues in children and adolescents. As we look ahead, ongoing research in child psychiatry promises to shed new light on brain development, the intricate interplay of genetic and environmental factors, and innovative treatment approaches. This article delves into these exciting areas of exploration and their potential for improving the lives of young individuals struggling with mental health challenges.

Advances in Understanding Brain Development

One of the most exciting frontiers in child psychiatry research is studying brain development in children and adolescents. Advances in neuroimaging techniques, such as functional magnetic resonance imaging (fMRI) and diffusion tensor imaging (DTI), have provided researchers with unprecedented insights into the developing brain.

Early Brain Development: Researchers are keenly interested in understanding how the brain develops during the critical early years of life. Studies have shown that early experiences, both positive and negative, can have a profound impact on brain structure and function. Investigating the mechanisms behind this plasticity could lead to interventions that promote healthy brain development.

Adolescence and Brain Changes: Adolescence is marked by significant changes in the brain, including continued refinement of neural circuits responsible for decision-making, impulse control, and emotional regulation. The research aims to uncover how these changes contribute to the vulnerabilities and resilience observed in teenagers, providing valuable insights for targeted interventions.

Exploration of Genetic and Environmental Factors

Child psychiatry research recognizes the importance of the complex interplay between genetic and environmental factors in the development of mental health disorders. Recent studies have made significant strides in unraveling these intricate connections.

Genetic Research: Advances in genomics have allowed scientists to identify specific genetic markers associated with various mental health conditions. Understanding the genetic basis of disorders like autism spectrum disorder (ASD) and attention-deficit/hyperactivity disorder

(ADHD) can lead to more personalized treatment strategies.

Epigenetics: Epigenetic research investigates how environmental factors, such as stress or trauma, can influence gene expression and contribute to mental health challenges. This area holds promise for interventions that mitigate the effects of adverse experiences.

Emerging Treatment Modalities

In the realm of treatment, child psychiatry is witnessing the emergence of innovative approaches reshaping how mental health conditions are managed.

Targeted Therapies: Personalized medicine is becoming a reality in child psychiatry. With a deeper understanding of the genetic and neurobiological underpinnings of mental health
treatments can be tailored to an individual's unique profile, increasing the likelihood of success.

Digital Mental Health: Technology is increasingly prominent in mental health care for children and adolescents. Teletherapy, mobile apps, and virtual reality interventions are expanding access to care and providing new tools for assessment and treatment.

Mind-Body Interventions: Research explores the efficacy of mind-body interventions such as mindfulness, yoga, and biofeedback in managing mental health conditions in children. These techniques promote self-regulation and emotional well-being.

As we peer into the future of child psychiatry, it is evident that ongoing research opens exciting possibilities for improved understanding, prevention, and treatment of mental health disorders in children and adolescents. Advances in brain development, genetic and environmental factors, and innovative treatment modalities offer hope and transformative opportunities for the well-being of our younger generations. Child psychiatry is poised to make significant strides in the years to come, enhancing countless children's and their families' lives.

Innovations in Child Psychiatry: Modern Treatment Approaches

Introduction

In the ever-evolving field of child psychiatry, innovations in treatment approaches are reshaping the way mental health conditions are addressed in children and adolescents. This article explores some of the cutting-edge advancements in the field, including technology-based interventions,
the rise of telehealth and online therapy options, and the growing importance of cultural considerations in treatment planning.

Technology-Based Interventions

Technology-based interventions have emerged as powerful tools in child psychiatry in an increasingly digital world. These innovations leverage the potential of smartphones, tablets, and computers to provide effective and engaging mental health support.

Mobile Apps: A growing ecosystem of mobile apps is designed to assist children and adolescents in managing their mental health. These apps offer features like mood tracking, relaxation exercises, and coping strategies, empowering young individuals to take an active role in their well-being.

Virtual Reality (VR) Therapy: Virtual reality is finding its way into treating conditions like anxiety and phobias. VR exposure therapy allows patients to confront their fears in a controlled and immersive environment, making it particularly useful for children and teens.

Biofeedback and Wearable Devices: Biofeedback devices and wearables provide real-time data on physiological processes like heart rate and skin conductance. These tools enable individuals to learn self-regulation techniques and manage symptoms related to stress and anxiety.

Telehealth and Online Therapy Options

The advent of telehealth and online therapy has revolutionized access to mental health care for children and adolescents, especially in underserved or remote areas.

Teletherapy: Teletherapy allows young individuals to connect with mental health professionals via secure video conferencing. This approach has proven effective for various conditions, including depression, anxiety, and ADHD. It also eliminates geographical barriers, ensuring that quality care is accessible to all.

Online Support Groups: Online support groups provide a sense of community and understanding for children and teens facing similar challenges. These virtual spaces allow for peer support, information sharing, and emotional validation.

Asynchronous Counseling: Some platforms offer asynchronous counseling, where clients and therapists communicate through messages or recorded video messages. This flexibility is especially appealing to adolescents who may prefer written communication.

Cultural Considerations in Treatment

Recognizing the cultural diversity within child psychiatry is crucial for delivering effective care. Cultural considerations encompass an awareness of cultural norms, beliefs, values, and the impact of acculturation on mental health.

Culturally Competent Care: Mental health professionals are increasingly trained to provide culturally competent care. This means tailoring treatment plans to align with their young patients and their families' cultural backgrounds and preferences.

Language Accessibility: Ensuring that therapy and resources are available in multiple languages and dialects is essential for reaching diverse populations. Language should never be a barrier to accessing mental health support.

Community Engagement: Collaboration with community organizations and leaders can help bridge cultural gaps and improve outreach. Culturally sensitive approaches build trust and enhance treatment outcomes.

Innovations in child psychiatry are transforming the landscape of mental health care for children and adolescents. Technology-based interventions, telehealth, and online therapy options expand access and engagement, while cultural considerations foster more inclusive and effective treatment approaches. The future of child psychiatry is marked by adaptability, accessibility, and a commitment to addressing the unique needs of every young individual, regardless of their background or location. These advancements pave the way for brighter, healthier futures for our younger generations.